Living With
A·I·D·S

*This book is dedicated
to Rachel, my beloved sister and inspiration,
and to the participants in the research.*

Living With
A·I·D·S

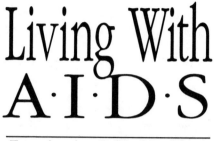

Experiencing Ethical Problems

Miriam E. Cameron

SAGE Publications
International Educational and Professional Publisher
Newbury Park   London   New Delhi

Computer graphics by Judith Leskela, St. Paul, Minnesota

For information address:

SAGE Publications, Inc.
2455 Teller Road
Newbury Park, California 91320

SAGE Publications Ltd.
6 Bonhill Street
London EC2A 4PU
United Kingdom

SAGE Publications India Pvt. Ltd.
M-32 Market
Greater Kailash I
New Delhi 110 048 India

Printed in the United States of America

Library of Congress Cataloging-in-Publication Data

Cameron, Miriam E.
    Living with AIDS : experiencing ethical problems/Miriam E. Cameron.
      p. cm.
    Includes bibliographical references and index.
    ISBN 0-8039-4778-X (cloth).—ISBN 0-8039-4779-8 (pbk.)
    1. AIDS (Disease)—Moral and ethical aspects. I. Title.
RC607.A26C34 1993
362.1'969792—dc20   93-25063
                                                CIP

93 94 95 96 10 9 8 7 6 5 4 3 2 1

Sage Production Editor: Yvonne Könneker

Contents

Foreword

Who can take away suffering without
entering into it?
                    Henri J. M. Nouwen, p. 72

Living With AIDS:
The Voices of Suffering

In no disease is the confrontation with personal finitude more direct, less compromising, or more insistent than in HIV infection. From the moment when a "positive test" is first announced, the person is caught in a maelstrom of suffering, the end of which—at least at present—is in all likelihood death. Yet, in the months or years before that end is reached, the individual must go on living. During the interval, family, friends, and the health professionals who attend the afflicted person also live unavoidably in a community of suffering, whose ethical challenges are among the most difficult humans are likely to confront.

For the person with HIV infection, suffering often begins long before the pain, the debility, and the dementia. On that account, it is all the more anguished, because for an extended time life seems the same and yet is not, nor can it ever be the same again. With a confirmed diagnosis of HIV infection, an existential barrier is crossed. If the caregivers are to help, they must somehow cross this barrier, too, to "enter into" suffering as Nouwen suggests. If they do not, or cannot, they may "do" many things for the person. But they cannot really help, because suffering engages the human spirit beyond the microcircuitry of the brain or the microphysiology of the body. The pain and symptoms of the troubled body must be mitigated, but this is not enough. To do this is only to stand on the threshold, but not to "enter" the individual's experience.

To "enter" the experience is exquisitely difficult. Each person's experience of suffering is unique. It is shaped by all those particularities of individual existence that give humans their personal identity. We can never completely enter into another's experience of illness. Paradoxically, however, *compassion* literally means "co-suffering." Compassion cannot exist unless we do enter to some discernable degree.

In this book, Miriam E. Cameron helps us to make the first essential steps. She takes us into the lived experience of persons with AIDS in the most effective way possible—by telling us their stories, which have remarkable powers of evocation. Each story teller speaks in her or his own "voice." To read each story is to share vicariously in the narrative of a particular individual's predicament of illness. These stories give us a privileged and intimate view of the values—ethical and other—that motivate these persons in their choices about how to live and how to die. Equally telling are the stories that relate the experience of family members and friends, who witness the suffering and must respond, each in her or his own way, to the desperate plight of their loved ones.

The persons whose stories are told here speak frankly and feelingly, but rarely bitterly, of their needs and how they are met, or not met, by the workings of the health care system or the professionals who attend them. Their ethical and spiritual doubts are laid bare as are the differences in their perceptions of what constitutes a "good" death. Significantly, requests for euthanasia and assisted suicide were rarely, if ever, included among the elements of a "good" death. What we have in so many stories is a rich and poignant insight into the spiritual and emotional odyssey these persons traced from their first awareness of affliction with this dread disease to the closing days of the drama of their lives and deaths.

Although some persons had formal religious commitments and others did not, all revealed the inescapability of the spiritual confrontation that comes with the certitude that one is marked for foreseeable death. Each in her or his own way struggled with Job's questions—Why? Why me? Why now? Why this way? All needed the understanding of friends, family, or pastoral counselors as they wrestled with these questions.

This is a volume of great importance to all who care for persons with AIDS. Here, starkly put, is the testimony of those we hope to help about the things they fear and recoil from, as well as the things that offer them solace. To "enter" suffering, we must seek to understand it from the sufferer's perspective and shape our treatment to that testimony. We are under an ethical imperative to resist reducing our care and caring to mere formula. It is impossible to stay at the threshold; we must, indeed, "enter" in a way that fits the uniqueness of the experience of suffering.

One comes away from these narratives not only with a vivid sense regarding the experience of these persons, but also with respect for their courage, honesty, and vulnerability. In their accounts, true compassion as co-suffering contrasts sharply with mere pity and sympathy, which are too self-serving and tinged with distance to be a genuine help to the sufferer. Indeed, to make the sufferer an object of pity and sympathy often only widens the distance and increases the suffering.

This book is an exemplary model of descriptive ethics, a branch of ethics still inadequately developed. Descriptive ethics details the values people actually use in making ethical choices. It provides the empirical data essential to the critical reflections of the normative ethicist and the metaethicist. These vivid vignettes about real persons uncover, in the most effective way, the personal nature of the ethical crises attendant on suffering and incurable illness. No lecture on ethical principles or theory can fully communicate what suffering is or what challenges it poses. Both principle and theory go seriously awry if they are not grounded in the phenomena so concretely described here. Without this grounding, normative ethics becomes a technical and dehumanized enterprise, too far removed from what humans think and feel.

Dr. Cameron, by virtue of her experience as a nurse and her special interests in ethics, is admirably suited to the task of linking these stories with the ethical issues they instantiate. She reflects in each chapter on the ethical problems these persons—and those linked to them—must confront about how to live, how to die, when to die, how vigorously to be treated, and when treatment becomes "futile." One need not accept the narrative theory of ethics, as I do not, to appreciate the significance for normative ethics of the living witness to what it means to be in confrontation with one's own finitude. This witness defines which principles and virtues are most crucial for those who genuinely offer to help.

These stories have much to teach all of us about living. We can learn humility from the way these persons confront challenges that dwarf our own responses to life's minor vexations. We learn, too, how many of these persons see the challenge of AIDS as an opportunity to grow in character and spirit. We see how even the gravest misfortunes can be an opportunity to sort out our values, to put them into an order so that they continue to give our lives new meanings and new value.

Clearly, as these stories show, health professionals must appreciate that healing can take place even with the sickest person. Healing means "making whole again." We may not be able to make the body whole again. But we can help those who suffer to continue to grow, to find meaning in life, even as it wanes; there is much healing that can occur even when death and decline are irreversible. These stories and lives contribute to the education of the human community in a unique way.

These stories also teach us something about ethical decision making. We can see that the complexity of moral decisions need not overwhelm us. The more awesome the decisions, the more need there is for thoughtful reflection and the more need there is to understand ourselves. Often we better define ourselves by our ethical choices in dire situations like these than we do in the lesser turmoil of everyday life.

Clinicians in all the health professions, ethicists, friends and families of persons with AIDS, and persons themselves with AIDS will find these stories immensely valuable. They provide the humane compass points that should keep our approaches to persons with HIV infection on course—clinically, ethically, and spiritually. These stories have much to teach about all manner of suffering—not only in AIDS, but in any tribulation. They have as much to teach about our own living and dying as they do about the experience of HIV infection. This is a contribution for which we owe much gratitude—to Dr. Cameron for allowing these stories to speak for themselves and to the persons whose voices we hear so eloquently enunciated in each story.

EDMUND D. PELLEGRINO, M.D.
Director, Center for the Advanced Study of Ethics
Georgetown University

Preface

Background

The roots of this book go back to my childhood when I sat in the corner of the living room listening to my parents and their friends discuss how they should bring up their children, make and spend money, and face illness and death. Years later, I realized that they had been describing ethical problems, situations involving conflict about the "right thing to do." Underlying their discussions had been their desire to resolve their conflict effectively about the right way to live and to die, perhaps the ultimate ethical problems confronting human beings.

While I was an undergraduate in nursing at the University of Minnesota, my professors explained that the goal of professional nursing is to benefit clients and that nurses should purposefully engage in activities that bring about this goal. I came to see that what these professors taught about nursing also applies to life. Both living and dying well can best be accomplished by purposefully engaging in behavior directed toward these goals, or behavior may only randomly, if at all, contribute to a good life and death. I wondered, however, what a good life and death were.

Later, I worked as a staff nurse, head nurse, nursing instructor, and hospital supervisor, during which time I experienced numerous ethical problems. For example, a child with cancer asked me why she was sick, and I questioned if I should I tell her the truth even though her parents had requested the hospital staff to say that a rare virus was causing her symptoms. Her parents had explained that lying was justified because talking about cancer would take away not only her hope but their hope as well. Sometimes, I lay awake at night agonizing about "the right thing to do" to resolve my conflicts.

As a nurse, I learned about good and not so good ways that people live and die. I became curious about what philosophers have written concerning living and dying well. Realizing that I lacked philosophical tools, I went back to school, completed a master's degree in nursing, and entered the Ph.D. program in nursing at the University of Minnesota.

Bioethics, ethics concerning health care, fascinated me, and I focused my doctoral work in this area. I completed a minor in philosophy and engaged in abstract discussions. Although I found philosophical ethics to be helpful and enjoyable, something was missing. Too often ethical problems were viewed as merely abstract, rational analyses, reflecting little of actual human experience. This kind of analysis lacked the contextual richness that I sensed was part of ethical decision making.

My coursework outside of philosophy and previous research experience had trained me to conduct quantitative research. However, the more that I learned about philosophical ethics, the more I turned to qualitative research and phenomenology, the study of phenomena or experience. I realized that phenomenology would provide an excellent conceptual framework and method for describing and examining the experience of ethical problems.

Ethics and Persons With AIDS

For my Ph.D. dissertation, I combined philosophical ethics and phenomenological interviews of persons with AIDS (PWAs) about their experience of ethical problems. Facing stigmatization and death, PWAs are forced to deal with dramatic, painful, and immediate ethical problems, rather than fix their attention on daily activities of living and avoid self-conscious recognition of the ethical implications of their choices. Furthermore, perhaps more than any other current disease, AIDS brings into focus the interaction between individual responsibility and societal responsibility for ethical living.

This book is based on my interviews with these PWAs and persons who were significant to them. Of course, no formulas are given about the right way to live and die, for living and dying are much too complicated. What the book provides is authentic stories from which you can glean understanding of your own ethical problems and, specifically, ethical problems involving AIDS. I hope that the stories will help nurses, physicians, therapists, other clinicians, ethicists, researchers, educators, and students to develop ethical clarity. In particular, I would like for the book to benefit AIDS-impacted persons.

In order to gain the most from the book, I encourage you to enter into a dialogue with the participants, with me, and, most importantly, with yourself. Some questions to ask are: In what ways are the participants' ethical conflicts similar to mine? What light do the participants' resolutions and rationale shed on my own resolutions and rationale? Why do I agree or not agree with the author's commentaries? What is the nature of my ethical problems? Finally, to what degree am I living ethically so that my resolutions to my ethical conflict and rationale for my resolutions lead to a good life and, eventually, a good death?

I reached out to the participants, and they generously helped me. I was kind to them, and they overwhelmed me with their kindness. Over and over, they told me that because of AIDS they now realized how "precious" life is. Facing mortality, they explained that they participated in the research so that their experiences would benefit other people and give them immortality. I hope that the book captures the essence of what they said.

Most of the PWAs who participated in the research have since died, and I feel a profound sense of loss. At the same time, I am grateful that they gave me the opportunity to experience the mystery of life and death, which is an incredible gift. They provided an ethics education by teaching me about living and dying well, most of which I cannot yet put into words. Because of the research, I may have had a small part in helping them and their loved ones to experience a good death.

A picture of a river is on the book cover. To learn about a river, some researchers would measure its length, width, and depth, whereas other researchers would examine a bucket of its water. This kind of research is similar to taking a bucket of water out of a river and analyzing its contents. During their interviews, the participants revealed a great deal about themselves. However, an interview is not a whole person any more than a bucket of water is the entire river. This metaphor also illustrates that just as a river keeps flowing when a bucket of water has been removed, life goes on for the remaining PWAs, for their loved ones, and for each of us.

Acknowledgments

This book would not be possible without assistance from many individuals. First, I am grateful for Michael Ormond, my beloved, nurturing husband. His emotional, intellectual, and financial support has never wavered. He has been my best friend, critic, and editor. Second, I wish to thank the PWAs and health care personnel who helped plan the research and recruited participants. Because of confidentiality, their names are not listed, but I appreciate their important contributions.

Third, faculty and staff at the University of Minnesota deserve appreciation for guiding the research, writing reference letters, editing what I wrote, and providing emotional support. Members of my Ph.D. dissertation committee were: Dr. Patricia Crisham, Dr. Verona C. Gordon, and Dr. Mariah Snyder (Nursing); Dr. Arthur L. Caplan (Philosophy, Surgery, and Director of the Center for Biomedical Ethics); and Dr. Douglas E. Lewis (Philosophy). Other helpful persons were: Dr. Janice Post-White and Dr. Muriel B. Ryden (Nursing); Dianne M. Bartels and Dr. Dorothy E. Vawter (Center for Biomedical Ethics); Dr. Mila A. Aroskar and Dr. Rosalie A. Kane (Public Health); Dr. Norman O. Dahl (Philosophy); and Dr. Frank S. Rhame (HIV Clinic Director). Dr. Cynthia Gross furnished an office for me, and Carol Reese provided instruction about interviewing skills (Nursing).

Fourth, I wish to express thanks for generous direct and indirect funding. The National Center for Nursing Research (NCNR) at the National Institutes of Health furnished an Individual National Research Service Award (F31NR06327) that paid for much of my doctoral education and the research. Dr. Doris Bloch, Dr. Patricia Moritz, Dr. Barbara Pillar, and Rick Wiener went out of their way for me. The University of Minnesota Graduate School provided supplemental funding with tuition fellowships and a grant for research expenses.

The writing of the book was funded in part by a Short-Term Fellowship in the Medical Humanities in the College of Medicine at the University of Illinois in Chicago. Dr. Timothy F. Murphy suggested how to revise my dissertation for a book, recommended appropriate literature, edited two drafts of the manuscript, and provided emotional support. Dr. Norman Gevitz, Dr. Barbara F. Sharf, and other faculty members made editing suggestions.

The Joseph P. Kennedy, Jr., Foundation and the Joseph and Rose Kennedy Institute of Ethics gave me scholarships to attend three intensive bioethics courses at the Joseph and Rose Kennedy Institute of Ethics, Georgetown University, Washington, D.C. Dr. James F. Childress, Dr. Edmund D. Pellegrino, Eunice Kennedy Shriver, Dr. Robert M. Veatch, and Dr. LeRoy Walters took a personal interest in my ethics education and the research.

While writing the book, I held positions, funded by federal and state money, at the University of Minnesota: Postdoctoral Fellow, School of Nursing Research Center for Long-Term Care of the Elderly, directed by Dr. Sue K. Donaldson; Center Associate, Center for Biomedical Ethics; and Faculty Fellow, Minnesota Area Geriatric Education Center, directed by Dr. Robert L. Kane.

Fifth, I wish to thank other colleagues and friends. Sue Hartman and Bridget McNeil accurately transcribed each interview audiotape within a week of the interview. Howard Bell, Dr. Felissa L. Cohen, Frank P. Lamendola, N. Holly Melroe, Dr. Susan D. Moch, Royce Nelligan, and Marjorie Schaffer provided expertise. Adrienne Bodor, Virginia Kivits, David Larsen, Ruthie LeDell, Mary Etta

Litsheim, Florence Littman, Jane Miller, Melba Miller, Leon Or-
mond, Elin Pederson, Meg Sandifer, Leila Texer, and members of
my ongoing Aristotle and philosophy discussion groups—Ray
DeVogel, Dr. Susan DeVogel, Deborah Dewalt, Donna Falk, Barry
Greenberg, Dr. David Jones, Dr. Joel Peskay, Vida Peskay, and Kate
Pfaffinger—offered emotional support. Finally, Dr. Diane K. Kjervik
introduced me to Christine Smedley, my editor at Sage Publications,
Inc., who understood and believed in the book.

   These persons contributed significantly to the strengths of the
book. Its defects are my own.

1

Overview

We all experience ethical problems, situations involving conflict about the "right thing to do." Some ethical problems are ongoing, such as conflicts about the right way to live and to die (Beauchamp & Childress, 1989; Frankena, 1973). Other ethical problems arise in specific situations. For example, a person with AIDS (PWA) confided to me, a nurse researcher, that he secretly used illegal drugs, engaged in unprotected sex with his girlfriend, and while claiming to her he was monogamous engaged in unprotected sex with other women. I wondered whether to maintain his confidentiality or let his girlfriend know about this behavior so that she could protect herself if she wished.

PWAs experience particularly difficult ethical problems because AIDS is life-threatening, communicable, chronic, and stigmatizing (Shilts, 1987). Often, PWAs are young, with little life experience upon which to draw when confronted by complicated ethical problems. How PWAs resolve their ethical problems can profoundly affect themselves, the people with whom they interact, their community, health care personnel, and society (Moritz, 1990). Although ethicists, researchers, and clinicians have written about ethical problems involving AIDS, research has not been published on PWAs' own experience of ethical problems.

The focus of this book is research conducted with 25 PWAs and 5 persons who were significant to them, referred to as significant

persons (SPs) (Cameron, 1991a). Their stories provide understanding of the experience of ethical problems, and in particular, ethical
problems involving AIDS. Major unanswered questions about
AIDS involve ethical problems: Why do some PWAs share needles
for injecting drugs? Why do some PWAs engage in unprotected
sex? Without answers, the best medical and public health measures may have little impact on AIDS. Only by giving precedence
to PWAs' experience can effective resolutions be developed to
ethical problems involving AIDS on individual, institutional, professional, and societal levels (Crimp, 1988).

AIDS

Acquired immune deficiency syndrome (AIDS) is a life-
threatening syndrome of illnesses attributed to the human immunodeficiency virus(es) (HIV). HIV infection ranges from asymptomatic infection to severe forms of the disease. Although clinical
presentation varies, HIV typically infects human T cells that are
essential to normal functioning of the immune system. With immune deficiency, the HIV-infected person becomes susceptible to
opportunistic organisms that normally would be harmless (Centers for Disease Control [CDC], 1987).

According to the 1987 definition of the Centers for Disease
Control (CDC), AIDS is characterized by HIV encephalopathy,
HIV wasting syndrome, or certain diseases due to immunodeficiency in a person with laboratory evidence for HIV infection and
without certain other causes of immunodeficiency (CDC, 1987).
The later 1992 CDC AIDS definition includes people who meet the
1987 definition and adds HIV-infected adults and adolescents
with CD4 lymphocyte counts under 200 (CDC, 1991b). This definition moves the AIDS diagnostic label earlier onto the disease
continuum, which is intended to be more inclusive of women and
injecting drug users (Chang, Katz, & Hernandez, 1992; Murphy,
1991d).

HIV disease is transmitted by sexual, parenteral, and perinatal
routes involving exchange of body fluids with an infected person.

Common routes include engaging in sexual intercourse with an infected person, using an infected needle to inject a drug, and receiving an infected blood product (CDC, 1992a). Life-style, environmental conditions, other viruses, drug abuse, and other cofactors can affect the progression of HIV infection. A person may be HIV-infected for many years before developing AIDS. Medications can inhibit HIV and help to treat opportunistic diseases (Flaskerud & Ungvarski, 1992; National Center for Nursing Research, 1990).

In the United States, most deaths from AIDS have occurred among people who inject drugs, men who have sex with men, and the sexual partners and children of these individuals. More Caucasians than people of color have died from AIDS. However, death rates from AIDS for African Americans and Hispanics have been higher than for Caucasians, resulting from their higher use of injecting drugs and subsequent HIV transmission to their sexual partners and children (CDC, 1992a).

Indeed, AIDS is a leading cause of death for some inner-city children and for women and men who are 25 to 44 years of age, surpassing heart disease, cancer, suicide, and homicide (CDC, 1992a). HIV disease rates are increasing among women, people of color, and persons who inject drugs. These increasing rates and higher death rates from AIDS for African Americans and Hispanics are associated with poverty, drug abuse, teen pregnancy, prostitution, child abuse, spouse battering, and inadequate education, health care, and social support (Bayer, 1989; Bell, 1989).

HIV infection is spreading throughout the world, particularly in developing countries, which have the fewest available resources for prevention and care (Earickson, 1990). The complex needs of HIV-infected persons are adding additional strain to already overloaded health care systems. In the absence of a vaccine or cure, effective educational programs appear to be the most useful tools for preventing HIV transmission (Blendon, Donelan, & Knox, 1992). The impact of HIV disease will depend on present efforts to prevent HIV transmission and treat HIV-infected persons (CDC, 1991b; National Center for Nursing Research, 1990).

Ethical Problems Involving AIDS

From a societal perspective, major ethical problems involving AIDS concern the right way to balance the public good with individual rights (Durham, 1991; Reamer, 1991; Whitmore, 1988). Most HIV-infected persons are people of color living in poverty and men who have sex with men. Even before AIDS, they were stigmatized by society. Fearful of AIDS, society blames persons with HIV disease for becoming infected. In particular, society has directed rage toward HIV-infected health care personnel (Lynch, 1992; Smeltzer & Whipple, 1991; Sontag, 1989).

Ethical problems arise because public health measures to control HIV transmission may limit the liberty and privacy of persons with or at risk for HIV disease and encourage additional discrimination toward them (Brooks-Gunn & Furstenberg, 1990; Friedman, DesJarlais, & Sterk, 1990). To resolve this conflict, most authors have recommended individual responsibility, with minimal societal, mandatory measures to limit HIV transmission. They have argued that other measures would be ineffective, costly, and unethical (Bayer, 1989; Bloom & Glied, 1991; Lovejoy, 1991; Stein, 1991; Stoddard & Rieman, 1990).

Other ethical problems that are addressed in the literature concern HIV-infected persons' right to health care, the nature of this health care, and who should pay for it (Almond & Ulanowsky, 1990; Bell, 1989; Daniels, 1990, 1991; Goldman & Stryker, 1991; Larson & Ropka, 1991; Moseley, 1989). Even with universal precautions, health care personnel frequently are afraid to care for HIV-infected persons (Alexander & Fitzpatrick, 1991; Campbell, Maki, Willenbring, & Henry, 1991; Forrester, 1990; D. Rogers, 1989), although research indicates that health care personnel may become less fearful when given accurate information (Armstrong-Esther & Hewitt, 1990; Brown, Calder, & Rae, 1990; Swanson, Chenitz, Zalar, & Stoll, 1990). Authors disagree about health care personnel's obligation regarding HIV infection. However, some professions, such as nursing, have issued policy statements about their ethical mandate to provide care without prejudice, unless the burden of care to the professional is greater than the benefit to the client (ANA [American Nurses Association] Committee on Ethics, 1988; National League for Nursing, 1988).

Summary of the Research

The purpose of the research was to describe and examine the content and basic nature of PWAs' ethical problems. The conceptual framework and method combined phenomenology and the three levels of ethical inquiry: descriptive ethics, normative ethics, and metaethics (Chapter 2). The 30 participants were 37% women and 53% people of color. They consisted of 25 PWAs and 5 non-HIV-infected persons who were significant to the PWAs and provided contextual understanding (Chapter 3).

During in-depth interviews, the PWAs described and validated 100 (45 different) ethical problems, and the significant persons described and validated 17 (16 different) ethical problems. Fourteen of the significant persons' problems were similar to the PWAs' problems, and 3 of them were new problems. To assure confidentiality, I changed a person's name in each ethical problem, so the 30 participants appear to be 117 persons. Ten content categories of ethical problems emerged, summarized in Table 1.1. Chapters 4 through 13 consist of the 117 stories about 48 different ethical problems, told in the participants' own words.

Three components made up the basic nature of the ethical problems. These components are illustrated in Figure 1.1 and examined in Chapter 14. Strategies emerged for facilitating ethical living, which results from a combination of individual and societal responsibility (Chapter 15).

After completing the participants' interviews, I interviewed the transcriber of the audiotapes for most participants. The Appendix consists of excerpts from her interview about how the research was affecting her view of the participants, AIDS, and ethics. Her struggle to verbalize her reactions may help you to put into words your own responses to the participants' stories.

Table 1.1 Alphabetical Summary of Content Categories of Ethical Problems Described in Their Own Words by 25 Persons With AIDS (PWAs) and 5 Significant Persons

ALCOHOL and DRUGS	• "Should I continue using alcohol and drugs for immediate gratification in spite of the long-term risk to my immune system?"
	• "Although I'm sober, should I go back to using IV drugs because of immediate gratification even if they damage my immune system?"
	• "Should I rob a bank to get money for drugs even though I may go to prison?"
	• "Should I give in to my craving for substances or continue with a happy sobriety?"
CHRONIC ILLNESS	• "Should I give in to despair about my deteriorating health or live as fully as possible?"
	• "Should I change my life-style so my health will not deteriorate so fast or continue as I have been living?"
	• "Should I live moment by moment or make plans for the future?"
	• "Should I continue to use expensive treatment that keeps me alive or stop using it and die?"
	• "Should I take dope (prescribed medication) to control my pain even though it isn't good for me?"
	• "How should I balance the needs of my children, my loved one with AIDS, and myself?"
DEATH	• "Should I give in to my fears about death or view death from a spiritual perspective?"
	• "Should I live the way that I feel like living or live in a way that will assure me of going to heaven when I die?"
	• "Should I commit suicide, which may be wrong?"
	• "Should I write a living will even though I do not want to think about my death?"
	• "How should I live fully while helping my loved one to experience a good death?"
DISCRIMINATION	• "Should I avoid people although I need them?"
	• "Should I be honest or secretive about AIDS?"
	• "Should I be honest or secretive about being gay and having AIDS?"
	• "Is it right to lie to avoid discrimination?"
	• "Is it right to be prejudiced toward homosexuals even though I believe in equality?"
	• "Should I tell travel authorities that I have AIDS even though they may discriminate against me?"

Table 1.1 Continued

FINANCE and BUSINESS	• "Is it right to engage in illegal activities to make ends meet?" • "Should I hold a job for financial and emotional reasons even though it jeopardizes my health?" • "Is it right to benefit from AIDS?" • "Although I value the expertise of lawyers, should I follow their advice when I don't trust them?" • "Should I plan a funeral I can't afford or be satisfied with a county-paid funeral?"
HEALTH CARE	• "Should I give up or fight to graduate from a nursing school that rejected me because of being HIV-infected?" • "Although I value the expertise of health care personnel, should I follow their advice when I don't trust them?" • "Although I value the expertise of health care personnel, should I follow their advice when they don't care about me?" • "Although I value the expertise of health care personnel, should I follow their advice that's unwise?" • "Although I value the expertise of my son's doctor, should I get another doctor who has a heart?"
PERSONHOOD	• "Should I believe in God and religion even though I have problems with them?" • "Should I be who I am or somebody else?" • "Should I be a good person or a bad person?" • "Should I keep going or give up?" • "Should I be accepting or angry?" • "Should I admit my powerlessness or try to control everything?"
RELATIONSHIPS	• "Should I have a child even though I have AIDS?" • "How should I balance my needs with my child's needs?" • "How should I balance my needs with the needs of my partner?" • "How should I balance my needs with the needs of my family and friends?"
SERVICE	• "Should I help other people or focus on myself?" • "How should I balance being an AIDS activist with a person with AIDS?"

Continued

Table 1.1   Continued

SEXUALITY	• "Should I engage in protected sex or unprotected sex?" "Should I be concerned about my partner's sexuality or focus on my own needs?" • "Should I accept or reject that I am gay?" • "Should I be sexual as a gay man even though I may infect someone with HIV?" • "Should I be sexual as a heterosexual person even though I may infect someone with HIV?"

Are the Participants' Problems Ethical Problems?

Some of you may not view the participants' problems as ethical problems. For example, why is conflict about what kind of funeral to have an ethical problem? True, the participants did not conceptualize their ethical problems according to principled thinking (Beauchamp & Childress, 1989) or ethical caring (Noddings, 1984), perspectives that dominate academic ethics (Chapter 2). Their method of ethical decision making was most like virtue ethics (Aristotle, 1987), which combines ethics, theology/spirituality, and psychology. They explained that underlying their conflicts were the age-old questions: What is the right way to live, and what is the right way to die?

During the pilot study, I first asked, "What situation involving AIDS has been most stressful for you?" Each person focused on stress. So I asked, "What situation involving AIDS has caused you the most conflict about the right thing to do?" If an individual was uncertain about the question, I asked, "Is there something that you have been lying awake at night worrying about whether you should do this or that?" Then the person said, "Oh, yes. I don't know what I should do about . . ." Throughout the rest of the research, I only asked the second question.

Even the participants who seemed to know nothing about academic ethics told me that they were concerned about "doing the right thing," whether or not they actually did what they said that they should do. They described their conflict, struggle to resolve

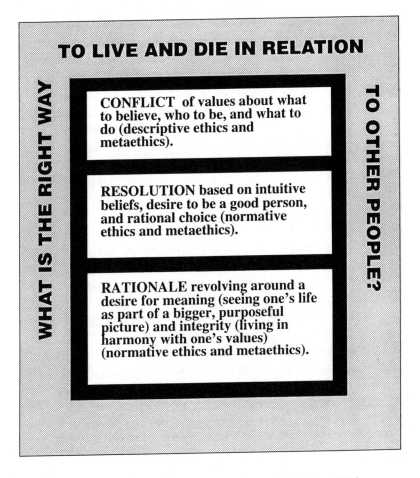

Figure 1.1. The Basic Nature of Ethical Problems Involving AIDS

this conflict effectively, and rationalization for the resolution. While talking, they frequently cried because of pain that they were experiencing from their conflict.

Because of confidentiality, I was not able to report an ethical problem in the context of the participant's entire interview. Otherwise, participants might be recognizable, and their stories could cause pain for themselves and their loved ones. Consequently, you cannot know that each participant's ethical problems were related and the underlying ethical problems were about the right way to live and to die.

During his initial interview, one participant described ethical problems concerning whom he should tell about AIDS, the right way to meet his sexual needs, and whether to be angry or accepting about AIDS. He had talked for nearly 2 hours when he said that he could draw better than talk. Taking a piece of paper, he drew the picture in Figure 1.2, explaining that conflict about the right way to live and die was the basis of his ethical problems.

This picture illustrates the underlying conflict for the other participants, too, whether they had been diagnosed with AIDS or were a significant person. Their presenting problems concerned whether to continue using alcohol and drugs, take prescribed medication, make out a living will, and other conflicts. However, the longer they talked, the more their conflict centered on the universal human struggle to live and die in the right way with some feeling of security in the midst of unpredictability, perhaps the ultimate ethical problems.

The question about whether or not the participants' problems are ethical problems may encourage debate, philosophical analysis, and empirical research. For this book, however, the question has already been answered. The participants themselves said that their problems were ethical problems, according to the definition that I gave to them.

Significance of the Research

Research indicates the importance of effectively resolving ethical problems (Cameron & Schaffer, 1992). For example, in various studies, nurses reported that ethical problems were the most stressful aspect of the job, in part because they were confused about how to resolve them. The more stress, the more likely nurses were to become "burned out." Burned-out nurses did not cope as well with ethical problems as nurses who were not burned out, and

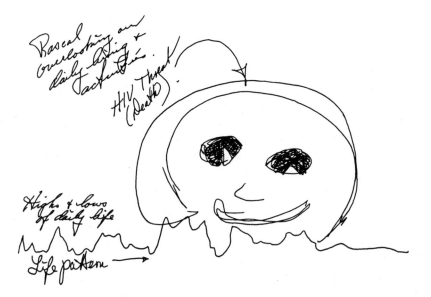

Figure 1.2. A Participant's Picture of His Underlying Ethical Problems Involving AIDS

NOTE: He explained that because of AIDS, he was walking down a "topsy-turvy" path with "highs and lows of daily life." He could see HIV, a "rascal overlooking our daily living and activities," constantly "leering at me," threatening death. Given the unpredictability of when and how "HIV will gobble me up," he asked, "What is the right way to live and the right way to die?"

they were almost six times as likely to have compromised their integrity, such as taking unauthorized work breaks (a form of stealing) and stealing hospital supplies and drugs (Cameron, 1986; Martin, 1990). If this research with nurses can be generalized to other people, help is needed first to understand and then to resolve ethical problems effectively.

Modern ethics education focuses on intellectual discussions in the Western philosophical tradition, which critics complain may offer little help for resolving actual ethical problems (Flack & Pellegrino, 1992). In contrast, the participants' real-life stories provide an ethics and AIDS education from a personal perspective and illustrate the variety of ways to resolve ethical problems. Because the participants' ethical problems are universal, anyone can identify with them, and the resulting elevated ethical consciousness may, hopefully, influence actual behavior for the better. A major strength of the research is the stories. I report each content category of ethical problems without interpretation. Only at the end do I describe my own views in the sections marked "Commentary." By using direct quotes and referring to other publications, I pull together the participants' descriptions of individual responsibility and societal responsibility in order to identify what can be done about the ethical problems described.

Another strength of the research is the participants' diversity. Until recently, most research has focused on Caucasian men and virtually ignored women and people of color (El-Sadr & Capps, 1992). Moreover, the five significant persons strengthened the research. Providing contextual understanding of the PWAs' ethical problems, the significant persons served as a reality check on the PWAs. This strength was most obvious when some male PWAs claimed to use condoms, whereas their non HIV-infected female sexual partners said that they did not use condoms consistently or at all. Finally, the numerous techniques to assure scientific adequacy strengthened the research by helping to accurately describe the participants' experience.

In summary, too often, society has created blank-faced stereotypes of PWAs. These stereotypes fail to acknowledge the specific, individual suffering accompanying AIDS (B. Rogers, 1989). The participants' stories put faces on ethical problems involving AIDS, as well as ethical problems in general, which can lead to effective resolutions on personal, institutional, professional, and societal levels.

2

Ethical Problems

At first glance, many of the participants' ethical problems may seem simple to resolve. For example, why question whether to use protection when engaging in sex? "That would not be an ethical problem for me," you might say. "Of course, I would use protection if I were HIV-infected because endangering someone else's life is wrong." While analyzing the participants' ethical problems, I came to see that they were much more complicated than I at first thought. Concerned that I was missing important components, I turned to philosophical ethics for help.

Philosophers have written extensively about ethical problems. True, their work has focused on philosophical analysis and, for the most part, has lacked empirical research about individuals' experience of ethical problems. Most published philosophers in the Western tradition have been Caucasian men, and their perspectives often have not been inclusive of women and people of color (Flack & Pellegrino, 1992). However, philosophers have made an important contribution by developing ethical theories that help to conceptualize ethical problems.

Ethical Inquiry

Frankena (1973) defined *ethics* as reflection on morality and *morality* as a social system of regulation that exists before and after the individual. While discussing their ethical problems, the participants engaged in ethical inquiry—investigation of situations involving conflict about "the right thing to do." Ethical inquiry occurs on three levels: descriptive ethics, metaethics, and normative ethics (Beauchamp & Childress, 1989), as illustrated by Sally's story.

Sally, a PWA, described conflict about her newborn, Nita, who tested positive for HIV antibodies. Although Sally wanted to be Nita's parent, she expressed concern that her daughter would develop HIV disease. She wondered if she would be able to take care of Nita while dealing with her own illness and possibly premature death. Should a good parent keep her daughter or let someone else adopt her?

When Sally discussed her conflict, she engaged in descriptive ethics, one level of ethical inquiry that consists of identifying characteristics of ethical problems (Frankena, 1973). Most previous descriptive ethics research has focused on hypothetical ethical problems rather than real-life ethical problems (Crisham, 1985; Rest, 1986). Much of the research has used Kohlberg's (1983) stage theory of moral development, which has been challenged for lacking relevance to women and people of color (Gilligan, 1982; Parker, 1990).

Sally engaged in normative ethics, a second level of ethical inquiry, by deciding the "right way" to resolve her conflict. Normative ethics consists of determining "right" resolutions to ethical problems. The essential premise is that some actions are morally superior to others and are for that reason choiceworthy.

By discussing the ethical term *good parent*, Sally engaged in metaethics, a third level of ethical inquiry. Metaethics consists of analyzing meanings of ethical terms such as *good person* or *right thing to do* (Beauchamp & Childress, 1989). Nurses and physicians do metaethics when they debate the meaning of terms such as *good nurse* and *good physician*.

As author, I am engaging in ethical inquiry, primarily with research rather than philosophical analysis. Using research to do ethical inquiry may be unfamiliar to some people, particularly philosophers. I engage in descriptive ethics and normative ethics by reporting the participants' ethical problems and suggesting how individuals and society should resolve them. When I analyze the basic nature of ethical problems and the term *ethical living*, I do metaethics. As a reader, you engage in ethical inquiry if the stories and my interpretations cause you to reflect on your own ethical conflicts (descriptive ethics), the right way to resolve them and why (normative ethics), and the meanings of the ethical terms that you use (metaethics).

Most published work involving ethical inquiry has revolved around normative ethical theories developed by philosophers. Because ethics is complex, one theory may not be adequate for all ethical problems. Each theory may reflect a specific domain, and certainly there are serious and sustained debates about the adequacy of any particular theory (Flanagan & Jackson, 1987).

Three major kinds of overlapping normative ethical theories involve principled thinking, ethical caring, and virtue ethics. Most normative ethics literature has focused on the perspectives of ethicists, researchers, and clinicians, rather than average individuals. In regard to AIDS, authors have primarily used principled thinking, and to some extent ethical caring, to analyze ethical problems. Authors have given little attention to virtue ethics, the kind of ethical theory that this research indicates can be important for resolving ethical problems involving AIDS, as well as ethical problems in general.

Principled Thinking

Principled thinking, which dominates academic ethics in the Western tradition, focuses on ethical principles such as autonomy and beneficence (Flack & Pellegrino, 1992). To resolve an ethical problem with principled thinking, a person would take a rational, impartial, impersonal perspective to analyze the problem using particular ethical principles, arrange the principles according to their importance, and select a resolution that accounts for each prioritized principle (Beauchamp & Childress, 1989). Associated theories are often called "justice" theories.

Some justice theories, called deontology, focus on the rightness of actions independent of their consequences. An example of deontology is Kant's Categorical Imperative. Kant (1986) used the principle of universalizability, which has been described as the Golden Rule without loopholes. The Golden Rule, "Do unto others as you would have them do unto you," allows mistreatment of other people if one does not mind being mistreated oneself. The principle of universalizability does not allow mistreatment because one cannot rationally will to be mistreated. Instead, the right action is what one can will for everyone else to do in a similar situation.

Alternative justice theories, called consequentialism, focus on the rightness of consequences independent of the actions that caused them. An example of consequentialism is Mill's utilitarianism (Smart & Williams, 1985). Mill used the principle of utility, defined as usefulness and doing the greatest good for the greatest number. In act utilitarianism, a right action maximizes the good. For rule utilitarians, an action is right if conformity to the rule under which it falls results in consequences that are at least as good as consequences of conformity to any alternative rule. An example of a rule is "tell the truth" (Smart & Williams, 1985).

Deontology and consequentialism are illustrated in answers to this question: Is it right to tell a lie that will bring about something good? A person who says that a lie is never right takes a deontological perspective, whereas a person uses a consequentialist perspective by saying that a lie resulting in good consequences is all right.

Most people account for right actions and good consequences when resolving ethical problems. Indeed, many philosophers have argued that a combination of deontology and consequentialism more accurately reflects morality than does one perspective. Beauchamp and Childress (1989), Frankena (1973), and Thiroux (1986) developed ethical decision-making models incorporating deontology and consequentialism, as illustrated in Table 2.1.

Table 2.1   Models for Ethical Decision Making Based on Principled
Thinking

Action Guides of Beauchamp and Childress

AUTONOMY	Be self-governing and allow other people to be self-governing; be my own person without constraints either by another person's action or by psychological or physical limitations.
NONMALEFICENCE	Do not inflict evil or harm.
BENEFICENCE	Prevent evil or harm; remove evil or harm; do or promote good.
JUSTICE	Give to another person his or her right or due.

Frankena's Mixed Deontological Theory of Obligation

BENEFICENCE	Do not inflict evil or harm; prevent evil or harm; remove evil or harm; do or promote good.
JUSTICE	Treat people as equals in the sense of distributing good and evil equally among them.

Thiroux's Universal Ethical Principles

VALUE OF LIFE	Revere life and accept death.
GOODNESS OR RIGHTNESS	Strive to be a good human being and attempt to perform right actions; try not to be a bad human being and avoid performing wrong actions.
JUSTICE OR FAIRNESS	Treat other human beings fairly and justly in distributing goodness and badness among them.
TRUTH-TELLING OR HONESTY	Engage in meaningful communication.
INDIVIDUAL FREEDOM	View all human beings, including myself, as individuals with individual differences and give them the freedom to choose their own ways and means of being moral within the framework of the first four basic principles.

Principled thinking, of course, has many critics. These critics claim, for example, that principled thinking reflects a restrictive, Caucasian, male, middle-class point of view and ignores the personal, virtue, and caring (Flack & Pellegrino, 1992; Fry, 1989;

Gilligan, 1982). It is unrealistic to demand total "objectivity" in the ethical domain, for human beings rarely, if ever, are impartial and impersonal about their own ethical problems. Moreover, no one determines the right thing to do about personal matters on a cognitive level alone. Instead of isolating abstract principles to resolve ethical problems, human beings look at ethical problems in context and take into account personal values (Blum, 1988; Condon, 1992). Principled thinking, critics argue, can reinforce existing power inequalities by producing ethical legitimization of the present system, not ethical evaluation of its values (Cameron, 1991b).

Ethical Caring

In response to criticisms of principled thinking, recent literature has advanced an ethic of caring. This theory has philosophic antecedents in Rousseau's teachings about compassion (Rousseau, 1979). From this perspective, a person will do the right thing about an ethical problem by feeling as nearly as possible what the cared-for feels and acting on the person's behalf in a concrete situation. Ethical caring necessitates an intuitive, empathetic, receptive mode arising from an ideal self developed in congruence with one's best remembrances of caring and being cared for (Fry, 1989; Noddings, 1984; Watson, 1990).

Instead of rationality as in principled thinking, ethical caring depends on a pre-act consciousness of relatedness, mutuality, and reciprocity (Condon, 1992). For proponents of ethical caring, the primary purpose of life is to care and be cared for, not obey rules or maximize the good. People who live according to the caring ethic will at least occasionally experience engagement, wonder, joy, and tenderness, despite pain, deprivation, and trouble (Cooper, 1991; Noddings, 1984).

Critics assert that ethical caring is inadequate for determining the right thing to do about complicated ethical problems. According to these critics, people will not be able to agree on intuitive approaches. Few people, after all, care for enemies or strangers. An excessive focus on caring may exploit women who traditionally have been expected to provide care in spite of inadequate compensation (Condon, 1992). Instead of encouraging a love of the good, caring may nurture a disproportionate love of that which is one's own. A caring person could act wrongly by being too personally involved with an ethical problem to make a good decision about how to resolve it (Cameron & Schaffer, 1992; Hoagland, 1990; Houston, 1990).

Although overlapping, justice and caring have distinguishing characteristics. Justice, which is associated with masculinity, consists of what one does, whereas caring, which is associated with femininity, involves who one is. Justice is abstract, objective, calculative, general, impartial, and impersonal, while caring is concrete, subjective, contemplative, particular, partial, and personal (Cameron, 1991b).

An integration of principled thinking and ethical caring may produce a more comprehensive normative ethical theory than either perspective alone. According to Aristotle (1987), both intellectual virtue (contemplative and calculative reasoning) and moral virtue (good character) are essential for ethical living. Frankena (1973) wrote that duty/principles and virtues/traits of character are not rivals but complementary to each other. Davis (1989) stated that ethical principles and virtuous character are necessary ingredients in ethics. Noddings (1990) acknowledged that justice may be needed in addition to caring.

To integrate these perspectives, Cameron and Schaffer (1992) developed the Caring and Justice Ethical Theory for use in clinical practice, as illustrated in Figure 2.1. A clinician can use this theory by analyzing an ethical problem from the perspective of each component in the theory, determine which components are most important, and develop a resolution that accounts for the prioritized components.

Virtue Ethics

Recently, some philosophers have argued that principled thinking and ethical caring describe only a partial view of morality, and

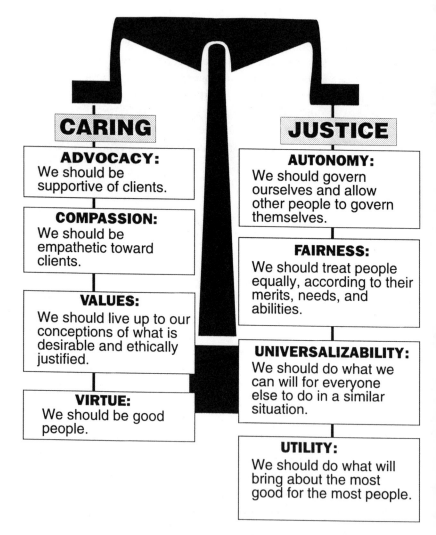

Figure 2.1. Caring and Justice Ethical Decision-Making Model

that a knowledge of virtue ethics can provide a more comprehensive understanding of ethical decision making (Pellegrino & Thomasma,

1988; Trianosky, 1990). Aristotle (1987) combined philosophy, theology, and psychology in what is called virtue ethics, and his writings continue to be the prototype for virtue ethics (Sommers & Sommers, 1989). According to this perspective, a person would "do the right thing" about an ethical problem by developing contemplative reasoning and moral virtue and then using calculative reasoning to resolve the problem.

Aristotle wrote that humans are rational and social beings. All intentional human activities aim at a good, and some goods are more important than others. The ultimate good for human beings is happiness, which means excellent functioning or virtue. Happiness is an activity, not passive amusement. In the highest sense, happiness is the contemplative life that is superior to other lives, and it includes friendship. Through education and habituation, humans can develop happy, virtuous lives.

Intellectual and moral virtue are essential for happiness. Intellectual virtue consists of contemplative reasoning and calculative reasoning. Contemplative reasoning is "an intuitive grasp of first principles," resulting in philosophic wisdom, and calculative reasoning is the rational determination of how to secure the ends of human life, resulting in practical wisdom. Moral virtue is excellent character or a disposition to choose the mean between excess and deficiency of a human behavior. For example, the mean between cowardice and rashness is courage.

Aristotle's virtue ethics includes the calculative reasoning of principled thinking and the intuitive, relational, compassionate mode of ethical caring. However, virtue ethics differs from principled thinking and ethical caring in major ways. Contemplative reasoning and moral virtue are central to Aristotelian ethics, not on the periphery, as in principled thinking and ethical caring. Without contemplative reasoning and moral virtue, calculative reasoning is blind because it says how to do something but neglects the meaning of doing it (Bishop & Scudder, 1990). For Aristotle, contemplative reasoning, moral virtue, and calculative reasoning are essential to effectively determine the right thing to do about ethical problems.

In summary, most authors have used principled thinking and ethical caring to analyze ethical problems involving AIDS, while ignoring virtue ethics. This kind of ethical analysis can leave out meaning and integrity, which the participants said was essential for effective resolutions to their ethical problems. The participants' method of ethical decision making was most like Aristotle's virtue ethics, with important implications for resolving ethical problems involving AIDS, as well as ethical problems in general.

3

Participants

Chapter 1 includes a summary of the research. However, some readers may prefer more details about the participants and the research process. For these readers, this chapter addresses who the participants were, the conceptual framework consisting of ethical inquiry and phenomenology, the method, and the ethical problems that I experienced concerning the participants.

Who They Were

Of the 30 participants, 8 women and 17 men were diagnosed with AIDS, 18 years old or older, physically and mentally capable of participating, and willing to participate. Besides the 25 PWAs, 3 other women and 2 men participated. If a PWA described an ethical problem involving a non-HIV-infected significant person who was at least 18 years old and capable of participating, I asked the PWA for permission to invite the person to be interviewed and provide contextual understanding, important in a phenomenological study. The 5 significant persons consisted of 4 sexual partners and a mother of PWAs.

I interviewed a heterogenous group of participants in order to elicit a wide range of responses to the phenomenon and reflect PWAs' diversity (Centers for Disease Control, 1991a). Furthermore, I wished to give voice to persons, such as women and people of color, who often are excluded from research and ethical discourse in the Western tradition (Dresser, 1992; El-Sadr & Capps, 1992; Flack & Pellegrino, 1992). Figure 3.1 illustrates the PWAs' mode of exposure to HIV infection, and Figure 3.2 indicates the race/ethnicity of the PWAs and significant persons.

The PWAs' ages ranged from 21 to 61 (average of 36), while the ages of the significant persons ranged from 22 to 64 (average of 41). The PWAs' education varied from fourth grade through postdoctoral work (average of high school plus 2 years), whereas the significant persons' education varied from high school through graduate work (average of high school plus 3 years). Although most of the PWAs said that they no longer worked full time because of discrimination or their deteriorating health, they previously had held a variety of positions. Seven PWAs, including two nurses, were or had been health care personnel.

In order to be respectful toward the participants while assuring the scientific adequacy of the research, I adhered to ethical standards for treatment of vulnerable human subjects and obtained a Public Health Service Confidentiality Certificate to protect their identity. I planned the research with PWAs and AIDS educators, interviewed participants whom I did not know, frequently consulted with various experts, and conducted a pilot study (Hall & Stevens, 1991).

Ethical Inquiry and Phenomenology

One component of the conceptual framework consisted of ethical inquiry, which I used to describe and examine the content and basic nature of PWAs' ethical problems involving AIDS, as follows: (1) descriptive ethics—characteristics of PWAs' ethical problems; (2) normative ethics—what PWAs said was the right way to resolve their ethical problems; and (3) metaethics—PWAs' meanings of ethical terms that they used, such as "right thing to do." The other component was phenomenology, the study of phenomena or experience (Spiegelberg, 1984), which I used to describe and

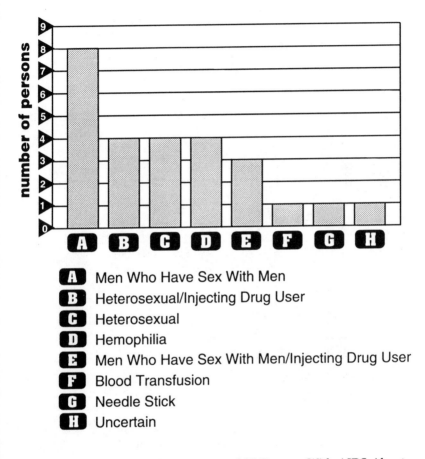

Figure 3.1. Self-Reported Descriptions of 25 Persons With AIDS About Their Mode of Exposure to HIV Infection

examine the PWAs' experience of ethical problems involving AIDS. Although a growing body of literature consists of phenomenological research, this perspective may not be familiar to some individuals, in particular to philosophers.

Phenomenological research is a type of qualitative research, research that produces words. In contrast, quantitative research yields mathematical characterizations (Sandelowski, 1991; Viney

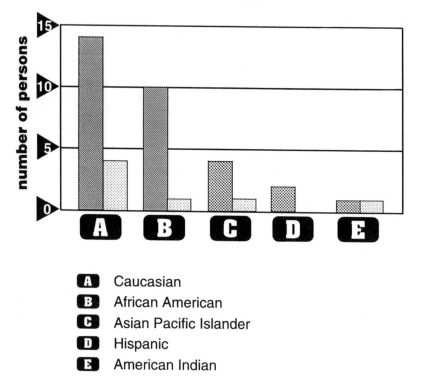

A Caucasian
B African American
C Asian Pacific Islander
D Hispanic
E American Indian

Figure 3.2. Self-Reported Descriptions of 25 Persons With AIDS (PWAs) and 5 Significant Persons (SPs) About Their Race/Ethnicity

& Bousfield, 1991). Phenomenological researchers interview participants about their experience of a particular phenomenon, and instead of imposing a framework on what the participants say, they allow essences to emerge (Oiler, 1986; Spiegelberg, 1984). In this research, the phenomenon in question is the experience of ethical problems involving AIDS, and essences are defined as the content and basic nature of the PWAs' ethical problems.

Method

Like the conceptual framework, the method integrated ethical inquiry and phenomenology. I used a three-step method based on work by Oiler (1986) and Spiegelberg (1984).

1. *Interview Participants:* Midwest health care professionals recruited PWAs, after which I explained the research, obtained written consent, and conducted an audiotaped interview of each participant. I asked, "What situation involving AIDS has caused you the most conflict about the right thing to do?" Using communication techniques such as "Uh-huh" and "Go on," I encouraged a full description of an ethical problem(s) involving AIDS and meanings of ethical terms used. Most interviews took place in the participants' homes and lasted from 1 to 3 hours. I conducted all interviews in person except for phone interviews of three PWAs and a mother of a PWA who lived in other parts of the continental United States and Hawaii, who were included to maximize racial/ethnic diversity.

2. *Analyze Each Interview:* I listened to the audiotape of an interview and then organized the interview into a verbatim outline of the ethical problems and their basic nature. To assure scientific adequacy, I conducted a second interview with each participant 2 weeks after the first one so that the person could correct and validate the written outline.

3. *Analyze Across Interviews:* Analyzing the content of the ethical problems, I eliminated repetitions, described each ethical problem in the person's own words, and identified emerging content categories. Next, I analyzed the basic nature of the ethical problems by describing commonalities and differences and eliminating repetitions. To assure scientific adequacy, five experts in AIDS, ethics, research, and phenomenology read all 30 outlines and two independent judges read randomly selected outlines to validate their consistency with the final analysis. No inconsistencies were reported.

Ethical Problems

Due to the nature of the research (C. Levine, 1991), I experienced five stressful, ongoing ethical problems. I turned to the literature for help but discovered that few authors have addressed ethical problems involving qualitative research (Fowler, 1988b; Ramos, 1989). Rather than struggle alone, I talked these problems over with colleagues to develop clarity about the right way to resolve them. My experience may stimulate debate about resolutions to these kinds of ethical problems.

One ethical problem was: What kind of a relationship should I have with the participants? I felt conflict between my values of being a good researcher and a good human being. To resolve this conflict, I abided by the contract between the participants and myself as stated in the written research consent form. I identified myself as a researcher and indicated with caring that our relationship would end after the second interview. Stepping out of my researcher role would change the terms of our agreement, I reasoned, which could be confusing and even hurtful to the participants and me. Only if a participant specifically needed my help was I justified in taking on a different role.

The participants made a variety of requests. After her second interview, a PWA asked if I would give her and her husband, who also had AIDS, a ride to their bank and home again. Another PWA requested that I help him to buy groceries with his "welfare check." I did what they requested because they said that no one else was immediately available to help them. A few weeks after her second interview, a PWA called me to ask if I would coauthor a book about her life. I encouraged her to write the book herself, and I offered to edit it.

A second ethical problem was: How should I be helpful, not hurtful to the participants? I felt conflict between my values of conducting good research and not hurting the participants. To resolve this conflict, I treated the participants with dignity by interviewing them where they were comfortable and paying any costs that they incurred, such as parking fees. I hugged them, held their hands, sat close to them, and took them seriously. After the second interview, I gave each person a flower to leave something beautiful in my place and a thank you letter containing an AIDS hotline number (after informing the hotline supervisor). By treating them with dignity, I reasoned, I could overcome any possible negative effects from the research.

A third ethical problem was: Is violating a participant's confidentiality justified to prevent harm to other people? I felt conflict between my values of maintaining the participants' confidentiality and preventing harm. The situation in which I felt the most conflict was when I interviewed male PWAs and their female partners who said that they were not HIV-infected. Each PWA told me that he usually used protection when engaging in sex with his girlfriend, but his girlfriend said that they rarely used condoms, if at all. Although each PWA told his girlfriend that he was monogamous, he told me that he periodically engaged in unprotected sex with other women and used illegal drugs.

I wondered if I had a responsibility to indicate my disapproval to the PWA and tell the girlfriend about the PWA's behavior so that she could take steps, if she chose, to protect herself from HIV infection. The couples seemed to be knowledgeable about HIV infection. In fact, one of the male PWAs said that he was so concerned about ethical problems involving AIDS that he served as a volunteer AIDS educator for teenagers.

To resolve this conflict, I identified myself as a researcher, not a therapist, and I did not offer advice or notify people whom the participants might hurt. Instead, I tried to understand without judgment what they said. So that each participant would grow in self-awareness and knowledge, I offered copies of the interview and analysis and brochures with information about AIDS. I reasoned that if I switched from being a researcher to a therapist, I might damage our tenuous relationship, and they might feel more alienated from society than they already seemed to feel and continue to engage in harmful behavior.

A fourth ethical problem was: Is violating a participant's confidentiality justified to maximize my safety? I felt conflict between my values of conducting good research and feeling safe. Many interviews took place in high crime areas and some PWAs had a history of violence and imprisonment. To resolve this conflict, I told my husband the location of an interview when I felt anxious about safety. I reasoned that I could ensure my safety by violating a participant's confidentiality in a manner that was not harmful. Fortunately, I did not experience safety problems. The participants were kind to me.

A fifth ethical problem was: What kind of person should I be in an unjust society? I felt conflict between my values of helping other people and looking out for myself. With each interview, I became increasingly and painfully aware of inequities in society. Sick, poor individuals, especially women and people of color, lack political and economic power. Often invisible to the majority culture, they primarily come into the public consciousness if they commit crime. I wondered if I should protect myself from the pain that I was feeling by becoming less sensitive to their difficulties.

To resolve this conflict, I kept in mind what was beautiful about the participants' lives, as well what was unjust. I resolved to give the participants a voice in this book in order to do my part about inequities in society. Living ethically, I reasoned, means being concerned not only about my own well-being but the well-being of other people. If each of us takes responsibility to live with meaning and integrity and contribute to society, we will create a better world.

In summary, the 25 PWAs and 5 significant persons who participated in the research consisted of 37% women and 53% people of color (African American, American Indian, Asian Pacific Islander, and Hispanic). Additional research and philosophical analysis are needed to effectively resolve the kinds of ethical problems that I experienced involving the participants.

4

Ethical Problems Involving
Alcohol and Drugs

Alcohol and drug abuse is an important factor in the transmission and development of HIV disease (Allen, Onorato, Green, & the Field Services Branch of the Centers for Disease Control, 1992). Substance abuse can damage the immune system, leaving the individual less able to combat HIV infection (Pfeiffer, 1992). Persons who abuse substances may engage in high risk sexual activities and share needles to inject drugs, which can transmit HIV disease (Steel & Haverkos, 1992). In the United States, new HIV infection is occurring most rapidly among persons who share needles to inject drugs, and their sexual partners (Grund, Kaplan, & Adriaans, 1991; Siegal et al., 1991).

The participants seemed knowledgeable about the link between HIV disease and substance abuse. Many of the PWAs said that they had a history of alcohol and/or drug abuse, from which they were making varying attempts to recover. These PWAs described difficult childhoods during which they were victims of sexual, physical, and verbal abuse from parents or other people who were addicted to alcohol and drugs themselves.

Figure 4.1 describes the participants' use of illegal drugs and injecting drugs, which included cocaine, Dilaudid, heroin, LSD,

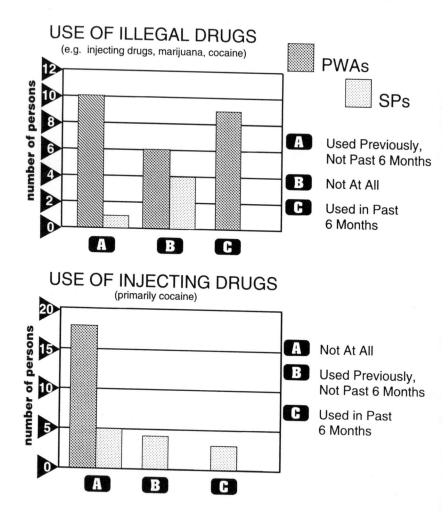

Figure 4.1. Self-Reported Descriptions of 25 Persons With AIDS (PWAs) and 5 Significant Persons (SPs) About Their Use of Illegal Drugs and Injecting Drugs

marijuana, mescaline, phenobarbital, speed, Talwin, and Valium, with cocaine and marijuana being mentioned most often. But the uses were not always escapist. Some PWAs, for example, said that they smoked marijuana for relaxation, relief from nausea, and appetite improvement.

Seven PWAs (three women and four men) specifically described ethical problems involving alcohol and drugs: "Should I continue using alcohol and drugs for immediate gratification in spite of the long-term risk to my immune system?" "Although I'm finally sober, should I go back to using IV (intravenous) drugs because of immediate gratification even if they damage my immune system?" "Should I rob a bank to get money for drugs even though I may go to prison?" "Should I give in to my craving for substances or continue with a happy sobriety?"

"Should I Continue Using Alcohol and Drugs for Immediate Gratification in Spite of the Long-Term Risk to My Immune System?"

JOE

Joe was a young, middle-class PWA at a small, Christian college, whom I met in a quiet room on campus so that his roommate would not know about the interview. He described conflict about whether he should use alcohol, marijuana, and LSD.

"If I might not be around a lot longer, why not use them for the immediate gratification that they provide?" Joe asked. "Should I give up immediate gratification because of the long-term risk to my not-so-top-notch immune system?"

Joe said that he was resolving his conflict by continuing to use these substances. Explaining his rationale, he said, "It's OK for me to use them to deal with AIDS. They help me out if I'm depressed because they provide immediate gratification. Their bad effects are long term, which I don't have to worry about because I may not be around that long myself." Pausing, he said, "I'm coming to realize that I should worry a little more about them. I'm 2½ years overdue, even though 3 years ago they said that I would only live 6 months."

CAROL

Carol and her husband, Pete, both had AIDS. Previously, they had been homeless, but recently the county had placed them in an inner-city apartment. As Carol and I sat by the kitchen table, she put her head in her hands. Like Joe, she described conflict about whether to continue using alcohol and drugs for immediate gratification even though they posed a long-term risk to her immune system. Her substance of choice was cocaine.

"Sometimes I need IV drugs just to make it through because life feels so unhappy," she said. "With HIV, it feels even more unhappy. But I'm scared to do them now. You hear if you do drugs, alcohol, you're taking more time off your life. I don't want to speed up the process. I want to live as long as possible."

"Maybe a reason for doing IV drugs is to block out death," said Carol. "I've been scared of death since being a kid. When I feel scared, I do drugs that for a little while take it away."

"They say once you're a drug user or alcohol user you never stop," she said. "But I have seen people stop. I stopped for 2 to 3 years. I went back, but I don't know why. Some people never stop until they kill themselves."

"I wonder why I do drugs," she continued, "because they don't last long. You want more. You don't feel the stuff. You're throwing money away. I get mad and say, 'Why did I do that?' I blame my husband. 'If he would have stopped me, I wouldn't have done it.' I blame my friends, and it's not right to do that, because I have control in my life. I let the drugs get control of my life, and that's bad. That uses up the money that I'd spend on food and other things."

Carol said that she had not resolved her conflict about whether she should use alcohol and drugs. "I may go back to IV drugs," she said. "If I got into them real bad again, I would probably steal money to buy them. Now I get money for drugs by doing tricks. Friends buying drugs come over. They buy for themselves and then share with me."

Explaining her rationale for using IV drugs, Carol continued, "I don't like to go to doctors, to take medication. Everybody says, 'How could you do IV drugs if you don't like blood drawn from

your arm?' Well, it's something different. The medical people take
something out. I'm putting something in. That makes a big difference. You're getting a different feeling."

"I don't know what would keep me from doing IV drugs," Carol
said. "I don't even know if I'd give them up if one of my children
died. There's nothing that doctors and nurses can do. They can't
hold your hand and watch you 24 hours. If they did, you'd get out
somehow and do them. They could sit and talk, but it's up to the
individual to stop. I'd stop doing drugs if I had something to live
for. I could say that time is running out so I'm not going to do
drugs because I don't want to speed it up. Only time will tell. I
can't say what the future might bring."

PETE

After Carol's interview, Pete walked into the kitchen. An AIDS
educator had told me about Pete's history of violence and incar-
cerations. I tried to put him at ease so we would both feel safe.
Like Joe and Carol, he discussed conflict about whether to continue using alcohol and drugs for immediate gratification in spite
of the long-term damage to his immune system.

"I don't much care for drinking," Pete began, looking at the
table. "I do it because I have pressure on me. It ease my pressure.
Get half-way loaded and don't bother me."

Pete said that he felt conflict about his drinking because it kept
him from eating. "I was hungry and sick. I come home. I made me
some liver and rice. I couldn't eat that. I got up and made some
early June peas. I ate a small amount of those and went to bed. I
get up this morning and ate me a couple of eggs. Eaten anything
since. But I hungry though." Moreover, Pete said that he felt
conflict about drinking because of the danger to his immune
system. "When they first told me about HIV," he explained, "they
said I shouldn't drink. Drinking didn't bother me then, but now
it kind of bothers me."

Also, Pete expressed conflict about whether to continue injecting
drugs. He said that they were not healthy, but he needed them to
engage in oral sex. "I'm a shy guy in sex," he said. "But if I get on drugs,

and I be with a woman, and she want to have oral sex, that's the only way I can go through with it. I can't do it otherwise. That's the only time I mess with drugs. I ain't never shot no drugs by myself."

Pete's resolution was to continue using alcohol. "I walk to the store and get me a half a pint of strong whiskey," he said, "and I sit here and drink and go to sleep. I don't get up till 8 the next morning. I wake up, I have a clear mind. Or buy a pint of dinner wine. Drink the whole thing myself. Or I go across the street and my buddy buy a half a pint. I dip in on that." Explaining his rationale, he continued, "My mind be more clear after drinking. Hatred go out of me."

However, Pete had not resolved whether to continue injecting drugs. "I have asked myself if I'd go back to drugs if I meet a woman I want to be with," he said. "I don't know. The last time I did drugs was a couple months ago. I was at a treatment center for chemical dependency. I did it there."

Explaining his rationale, he said, "Being HIV doesn't make any difference in deciding whether to do drugs. If I feel like doing drugs, I'll do them. I would share dirty needles if I didn't have clean ones. I could get money for drugs. I've been in the penitentiary 13 times for forgery, theft, burglary, receiving stolen goods, but I wasn't always caught."

"Although I'm Sober, Should I Go Back to Using IV Drugs Because of Immediate Gratification Even if They Damage My Immune System?"

BETH

Because Beth, a PWA, was concerned about confidentiality, I interviewed her at an agency with the lights turned low so that we could not see each other very well. She explained that she had been sober for almost a year but expressed conflict about whether to inject drugs again.

"When I learned about being HIV-infected," Beth began, "I decided to go for treatment and lasted a week. I figured that getting high was better because I was going to die, and I might as well die high. The last time I used IV drugs I was sick because I had caught pneumonia when I was running around in a sweat jacket in 30 below zero weather because I thought it was summer. If I kept this up, I'd get sicker. I told them that I'd go to treatment if I got to choose the place. It took me four times through treatment to quit using."

However, Beth wondered if she should go back to injecting drugs again. "I enjoyed getting high. I was used to it. I started using IV drugs when I was 13. That was the only way I knew how to get by. I was able to talk to people and have friends. All my friends were users. They were like family to me. It's hard to avoid those old situations. I crave IV drugs when I see them or am around old friends."

Beth was resolving her conflict by not injecting drugs, for now. "My roommate's sober, and we stay away from situations of using," she said. For awhile, she maintained her sobriety by participating in Alcoholics Anonymous, although she did not go to meetings as much any more. She rationalized, "Using was ruining my health. I want to stay alive, I don't want to die. It would be stupid for me to use because it would break down my immune system and kill me. The more I'd use, the sicker I'd get. At times, I wish I'd never started drugs. Who's to say if I would have HIV now. I tell myself, 'That's stupid. Why worry about the way things could have been? You can't change what happened.' Instead of feeling guilty, I concentrate on today."

JANET

After the interview, Beth gave me a hug and left. Then Janet, her lover and a PWA, walked into the room. Janet said that she had been sober for 4 months. Like Beth, she described conflict about whether to go back to injecting drugs.

"I quit and then found out that I was HIV positive," Janet said, "and I started using again. It got to the point where I needed to stop because of my health status, finances, and job. I'm miserable when I'm using drugs. I'm not happy, and no one's happy with me. When I'm sober, people want to be around me. But I crave drugs because they helped me escape from the worst tragedy of my life—HIV. My partner didn't care if I stopped doing drugs. I quit working because of AIDS and had nothing to do. Drugs filled up the time."

Janet, like Beth, was resolving her conflict by not injecting drugs, for now. "My partner and I stopped doing drugs," she said. "I went into a half-way house and got a lot of support not to do drugs. I've had a few relapses since then. I stay sober by steering clear of situations where I might use drugs. I changed my friends, so I don't have many friends who use illegal drugs. I go to AIDS support groups, but I don't go to AA because it bores me. I get support from friends."

Explaining her rationale, Janet said, "I need to be sober because I'm an addict. Doing drugs isn't going to make me live any longer. If I was around friends who were using, then I'd for sure use, too. If I even see coke, I'm going to use it. I don't think I'll ever be strong enough to ignore coke if someone offers it to me. So I have to avoid the situation."

"Should I Rob a Bank to Get Money for Drugs Even Though I May Go to Prison?"

TED

Ted, a PWA, no longer used drugs, but he was considering going back to them. His conflict differed from that of Beth and Janet. Ted had robbed banks to pay for drugs. Eventually, he had been caught, convicted, and sent to prison for many years. Because of AIDS, his health was poor. His friends were able to get him out of prison so that his family could take care of him at home. Even after many years of sobriety, though, he craved drugs. He wondered if he should rob another bank and risk going back to prison in order obtain enough money for drugs.

"I used to do heroin and cocaine," Ted began. "It's one of the greatest things. I robbed several banks over the course of my career as a bank robber to get money for drugs. I robbed them because that's where the money is. I got a whole bunch of money." He said that he wanted to rob another bank to get money for drugs but he was afraid of going back to prison.

"I used to work for a national bank," said Ted, explaining how he became a bank robber. "The man who owned the bank was very rich, and I felt that he should share. The FBI or Treasury Department told us ways to identify phony identification. They said the bank is insured. We don't need any heroes. Just give them what they want. But I knew if you robbed a bank you'd go to prison."

After Ted robbed several banks, the authorities sent him to prison. "I stopped using drugs in prison because the availability ran out," he said. "In prison, I didn't get good medical treatment for AIDS. Why I didn't die I don't know, probably because of my positive will to live. I'd still be there except that friends helped me get out. I wanted to be with my parents and get some top-notch medical care, and that's what happened."

At home with his parents, Ted was resolving his ethical problem by not using drugs anymore. Then he no longer needed to rob banks to pay for them. In describing his rationale, Ted said that robbing banks was not wrong for him. "You didn't need a gun. All you needed to do was talk or give a note. I never wanted to hurt anybody. I've never hurt anybody with a weapon."

He explained why he no longer used drugs. "I don't use drugs now because I don't want to go to prison," he said. "If I do drugs or rob banks, I'll go back to prison. Prison is not a nice place to live, and I never want to go back. I got tired of smelling men's body odor and seeing the same people every day. You have fun, you don't walk around crying. But I hate whiners, and this serial killer was a whiner. He'd turn off the TV, which was irritating. I've never taken freedom for granted. When they hospitalize me, I hate it even though it's for my good."

"Should I Give In to My Craving for Substances or Continue With a Happy Sobriety?"

DANIEL

Daniel, a PWA, was well educated and lived in a trendy apartment. Sitting on the couch, I looked at art on the wall and heard classical music in the background. He said that although he had completed 2 years of "happy sobriety," he felt conflict about the right way to deal with his craving for substances.

"At age 10," Daniel began, "I started abusing mind-altering substances. I wasn't what I wanted to be, and they filled the void. I was arrested for buying and selling drugs, and I accumulated thousands of dollars in debt and hot checks. Before college graduation, I was diagnosed with HIV. I figured it was God's punishment for a life-style that was not the way a man should live. I didn't want to live or die, so I became more abusive. I felt guilty because I was alive and for engaging in unprotected sex. I thought I had caused some people to die from AIDS. After snorting heroin and doing speedball, I would get on my knees and say, 'Please, God, take this away,' knowing that I would go back to using."

He went on, "My parents unknowingly enabled me. They said, 'You don't have a drug problem.' I have this incredible knack of manipulating people. But they finally got through. It hit me like a whirlwind that I couldn't do drugs anymore. 'I'm alive for a reason. For 5 years, I've lived with this virus even though I was supposed to die from it. I need to find out what life's about.' Divine intervention had a lot to do with it."

Daniel resolved his conflict by going through treatment twice. To experience a "happy sobriety," he participated in Alcoholics Anonymous and other support groups, and he worked as a "volunteer AIDS and chemical addiction educator."

"I'm learning to like and be responsible for me," Daniel explained. "Abusive behavior isn't an option because I want to live. I can't know what tomorrow will bring. I have to make the best of today. There's much to grasp, to recognize, to be blessed by. I am here for a reason, to make a difference, not just for myself, but for people whose lives I can touch. The universe is abundant, and somewhere I fit into the scheme of things. The serendipity of it all, the gift is me. Previously, I thought the gift was material things or a person."

Daniel told a story. "One day when my grandfather was walking me to kindergarten, I jumped into traffic because the street sign said walk. He pulled me up on the curb and scolded me, and I began to cry. He told me a car was turning around the corner and wasn't looking at the walk sign. He said to watch the cars, because the light never hit nobody. He was saying, 'There's more to life than what's in front of you. Things to the side, behind, all around you can be threats or helpful.' His wise words help me to have a happy sobriety."

"To become sober meant dealing directly with who I am instead of running away," Daniel continued. "Life is fearful whether or not you use. Without drug use, the possibilities have been limitless for me. I've made dear friends. I know that people care, and I can give to them. HIV has turned out to be positive in my life. If people choose to accept what they are, they can move through anything and find out that it is a blessing. God as you understand Him will come into your life to let you realize His will be done. Different things are put in people's lives to let them see there's something more than what we know to make life worth living."

Commentary

The stories of the seven PWAs who described ethical problems involving alcohol and drugs dramatically illustrate how feelings of hopelessness, despair, and alienation can lead to and accompany substance abuse, buying and selling drugs, and obtaining money for drugs through stealing and prostitution. Although the PWAs said that they were concerned about substances aggravating their health problems, they nevertheless craved substances for "immediate gratification" to help them cope with their prolonged unhappiness and anxieties about death.

The link between AIDS and substance abuse has created difficult ethical problems for society. These problems have revitalized the public debate about drug policy and the appropriate role of the government in regulating the behavior of competent adults (Decker, 1987). Proponents of drug decriminalization argue that drug use does not necessarily lead to dependency and dysfunctional behavior, and that decriminalization would reduce the counterproductive consequences of huge expenditures on repressive measures (Winick, 1991). Critics contend that decriminalization would encourage drug abuse, which could contribute to HIV transmission and cause even greater problems for individuals and society (Bayer, 1991a).

The PWAs did not indicate if a diagnosis of AIDS amplifies or lessens substance abuse. Some PWAs said that they became sober after learning about their diagnosis, but other PWAs used substances to cope with it. However, their stories provide evidence that substance abuse can lead to risky behavior and other difficulties. Pete engaged in sex while injecting drugs. To obtain money for drugs, Carol worked as a prostitute and spent her "welfare" money that was to be used for food. Ted had robbed banks, and Daniel had sold drugs and passed bad checks. Pete and Carol did not consistently use condoms, and Pete used "dirty needles" if clean ones were not available.

Ethical problems involving substance abuse are particularly difficult to resolve because alcohol and drugs can contribute to people's happiness, as well as unhappiness. Joe asked, "If I might not be around a lot longer, why not use them?" For Carol, drugs "put something in," helped her "to make it through because life feels so unhappy," and let her "block out death."

To reduce substance abuse and thereby curb HIV transmission, federal and state governments have substantially increased funds to expand publicly funded intervention programs, with some positive results (Chitwood et al., 1991). However, these programs have too few openings for the number of persons needing and wanting them (Boyle & Senay, 1991). Furthermore, workers in these programs often do not have training in both AIDS and ethics (Ashery, 1992; Calsyn, Saxon, Freeman, & Whittaker, 1992; McCusker,

Stoddard, Zapka, et al., 1992). Even if such programs become more readily available, questions arise about where to offer them, who should pay for them, how to provide counseling and testing, and what interventions are effective (Blanchet, 1990; O'Neill, 1987). Pete, for example, said that even when he was in treatment for substance abuse he had continued to inject drugs.

One controversial approach used to reduce HIV transmission resulting from substance abuse consists of giving addicted persons, such as Carol and Pete, clean equipment for injecting drugs and teaching them to sterilize their old equipment (Karpen, 1990; Primm, 1990; Staats, 1992; Stryker, 1989). Some research indicates that persons who inject drugs accept and absorb the educational messages of these programs, and they modify their behavior to avoid the risk of HIV transmission (Obermeyer & Streeter, 1991). Additional research and evaluation are needed to determine the effectiveness of these programs (Hartgers, van den Hoek, Krijnen, & Coutinho, 1992).

Instead of focusing almost exclusively on persons who actively abuse substances, more of society's resources could be directed toward people who are trying to stay sober. Innovative programs could be developed to help individuals experience a "happy sobriety" (to use Daniel's words) so that they have less of a need to go back to substance abuse. Certainly, these programs need to take into account cultural, political, and racial aspects of drug use (Friedman et al., 1990).

Additional programs could be developed in which former substance abusers function as community health workers for helping persons who are presently abusing substances or are new to recovery (Cooper & Weiss, 1989). Daniel said that he served as a "volunteer AIDS and chemical addiction educator." Other persons with a history of substance abuse might find similar activities to be helpful in staying sober.

Programs concerning substance abuse need to address the needs of children as well as adults. The PWAs told me that they began using alcohol and drugs during childhood to cope with physical, mental, and/or sexual abuse. "I started using IV drugs when I was 13," said Beth. "That was the only way I knew how to get by."

Effective strategies to prevent and curb substance abuse need to be developed for use in grade school, high school, and post-secondary education.

The PWAs' stories illustrate how some people take individual responsibility to maintain their sobriety in difficult circumstances. As Janet put it, "I stay sober by steering clear of situations where I might use drugs. I go to AIDS support groups." Daniel said, "I'm learning to like and be responsible for me. To become sober meant dealing directly with who I am instead of running away. There's something more than what we know to make life worth living."

In summary, the PWAs suggested how individuals who abuse substances can become and stay sober. However, society also has responsibility to prevent and curb substance abuse (Poku, 1992). Although the choice to live with meaning and integrity is the responsibility of the individual, social conditions that lead to hopelessness, despair, and alienation can make this choice difficult.

5

Ethical Problems Involving Chronic Illness

Like other chronically ill individuals, PWAs often do not know how they will feel from day to day. Severe illness may be followed by periods of wellness, or vice versa. Opportunistic infections present a range of clinical symptoms that require a broad repertoire of interventions (Cohen, 1991; Levine, 1990b). The PWAs described symptoms that they were experiencing, including "fatigue," "dementia," "medication reactions," "night sweats," "pain," "rashes," "thrush," "diarrhea," "weight loss," "retinitis," and "seizures." Some PWAs said they were under the care of physicians. Other PWAs explained that they did not trust the health care system, and they were treating their symptoms themselves or using approaches such as spiritual healing.

Eight PWAs (two women and six men) and two significant persons (women) specifically described ethical problems involving chronic illness: "Should I give in to despair about my deteriorating health or live as fully as possible?" "Should I change my life-style so my health won't deteriorate so fast or continue as I have been living?" "Should I live moment by moment or make plans for the future?" "Should I continue to use expensive treatment that keeps me alive or stop using it and die?" "Should I take dope (prescribed medication) to control my pain even though it isn't good for me?" "How should I balance the needs of my children, my loved one with AIDS, and myself?"

"Should I Give In to Despair About My Deteriorating Health or Live as Fully as Possible?"

MARY

Although Mary, a PWA, was nearly blind, she said that she took care of her husband, who also had AIDS. He lay in the bedroom as Mary and I talked in the living room of their home. She questioned whether to give in to despair about her and her husband's deteriorating health or live as fully as possible.

"What worries me is my eyesight," said Mary. "I lost most of my vision because of diabetes. I love to cook, clean, take care of the home and my husband. Not having my vision bothers me. I worry about what's going to happen to me when my husband dies. He hopes nobody takes advantage of me because I am too kind to people. To not be together will be lonely. How will I do things? When I see blind people get around, I don't think I can do it. It's scary. I've lived a good life, been monogamous, married, and I haven't used IV (intravenous) drugs. Why have I ended up with AIDS?"

Describing her resolution, Mary said, "We got to accept and go on. Be fighters. I'm not bitter. I'm seeing enough to have a clean home, cook food, and take care of my husband and myself. I have the Bible on tape, so I listen to it and the radio station for the blind. I pray, go to church and a support group, and I reach out to people. I encourage and inspire. Discrimination or whatever we're faced with, I don't dwell on it."

Mary explained her rationale. "You have to accept and go on with your life," she said. "From church and my support group, I get strength and connectedness with people and God. It's easier to face problems with support. When you let out how you feel, people can reach out and help you. I don't believe in telling the neighbors. But you have to trust somebody. Who knows, God may give them the right words to say to you."

"When you have inner peace, you can face anything," Mary continued. "It's not one day and tomorrow you angry and bitter. When you hear other people's problems, you can reach out to them so they don't make the same mistakes you did. You forget your health problem. I'm praying that they find a cure for AIDS. My goal is to see people educated. Life is precious. If people don't do destructive things, they live happier."

JOHN

Because John lived more than a thousand miles away, I interviewed him over the phone. I included him to reflect the racial/ ethnic diversity of PWAs. He said that he was diabetic and had developed AIDS-related dementia, although he spoke clearly during the interview. Like Mary, he questioned whether to give in to despair about his deteriorating health or live as fully as possible.

"I'm limited in my activities," John said vehemently. "I hate AIDS. I don't want to be restricted. I want to be free to do what I want. AIDS is keeping me from doing that."

"In small ways," John said, describing his resolution, "I'm trying to live so I feel like I'm a part of life, despite my problems. I am living my life in a different way because of AIDS, but I'm in there fighting to be as normal as I can." He rationalized, "I want to live a normal life because it beats living an abnormal life."

JACKIE

John lived with Jackie, his mother and a significant person. During her interview, she focused on her son's situation, not her own, as she described conflict about whether she should give in to despair about his deteriorating health or help him to live as fully as possible.

"Watching a child die is the most painful thing that can happen," Jackie said tearfully. "They are going to go, and you will be here. It doesn't seem right. A parent is supposed to die first and then a child. What's so frightening is that he won't be there anymore. He's going to miss so much. He said, 'Mom, I've lived a wonderful life. I've enjoyed music, art, nature, horseback riding.' That gives me comfort. I imagine that he hasn't missed much. But the idea of him not having a full life is frightening. Even though he's sometimes taken the wrong bend in the road, he's also had so much potential."

"What do I do to make his life happy and normal?" asked Jackie. "You're floundering each step of the way. What is the right thing? What is the wrong thing? What can you expect next? Your life changes totally. It's put on hold. Your whole being is devoted to taking care of your child. Your relationships with people are changed. Your relationship in the family is changed."

Describing her resolution to her conflict, Jackie said, "I quit my job to take care of him. I took classes on home care, and I learned about symptom management. I looked for community resources. Knowing what to do makes it easier. For example, a seizure is frightening. They explain what happens and how to handle it."

"I am responsible," said Jackie, explaining the rationale for her resolution. "My code of ethics can't change because of AIDS, or I wouldn't be who I am. There are things that give life meaning. You have to care, nurture, love, give. If you don't do that, why live? That's what my code of ethics is. A code of ethics is instilled by your upbringing. It's part of being a human being to live by your code of ethics. If I let him down, it wouldn't be devastating for him as much as my code of ethics."

"One must have quality," Jackie continued. "Otherwise, there's no point to living. It's not how long you live but what kind of a life you have while you're alive. Quality life means being loving, caring. You can make life good and happy, in spite of everything. To be able to enjoy what you can, give what you can give. Because the opposite kind of life isn't worth living."

"Should I Change My Life-Style so My Health Won't Deteriorate so Fast or Continue as I Have Been Living?"

MATTHEW

Because Matthew was concerned about confidentiality, I interviewed him secretly in the back room of an agency, rather than in his home. He told me that as a young, gay man of color, he had experienced discrimination. To avoid additional pain, he did not want any more people than necessary to know that he had AIDS. He appeared to be healthy, but 2 weeks later he was seriously ill in the hospital. At his invitation, I conducted his second interview at his hospital bedside.

During the first interview, Matthew questioned whether to change his life-style so his health would not deteriorate so fast or continue as he had been living. "It's hard to go from one extreme to the next," he said. "It's scary because of how vulnerable the body is to various diseases. I might not live a long life. It's scary to be young and have a disease that can take over. There are things that I shouldn't do anymore."

"I have to live with the changes in my health," Matthew said about his resolution to his conflict. "I no longer smoke cigarettes because of complications that I might suffer. I eat right, get rest, and exercise. Have a good relationship with my doctor and caregivers. I'm more cautious because of AIDS, how I approach the subject with various people, how I think about life itself. I try to excel in what I do and make things like school, my job, my family, the friends I have left a priority."

Describing his rationale for his resolution, Matthew said, "It's important to take care of my body. I take AIDS into consideration. You have to learn to live with the changes. You don't know from day to day if your situation is going to be good or worse. We take for granted how fragile and important life is. I'm young and I have a lot to live for. So I want to be around as long as I can and be healthy and be able to enjoy and endure the things that life has to offer. Be able to go to work, do recreational activities, travel."

JIM

Because Jim wanted to meet me before inviting me to his home, the first interview took place at an agency. The second interview was in his apartment. Like Matthew, he described conflict about whether to change his life-style so that his health would not deteriorate so fast or continue as he had been living.

"Everything's become such a rush," Jim said. "You thought you was going to live a long time, and you wasn't going to have complications to prevent you from doing what you want to do. You tend to become anxious about fulfilling your dreams. Should I change my life, my eating habits, and sleeping habits? Should I stop doing IV drugs and practice safe sex? Can I have a less hectic life than I do now?"

"The plan is to prolong your ability to do for yourself," Jim resolved. "Those negative habits you had, you drop them. Everything becomes more positive. You change your eating habits, your sleeping habits. You reserve your energy. I relocated because of stress. You try to relive sections of your life that you missed because of using IV drugs."

"Life is worth living," Jim rationalized. "You can arrange your life in a peaceful manner. This brings out a more serene, good feeling inside. I didn't have respect for life, because if I did I wouldn't be using IV drugs, and I would practice safe sex. AIDS makes you more aware. The dreams I put off have become relevant. You have death at arm's reach, lurking trying to get at you."

"By making changes," Jim said, "I want to put off death because I don't feel like I've accomplished anything. I haven't taken seriously to help other people because I always thought that people retire when they're 60, and then they reach out for other people. I'm starting to realize I need to be doing that all the time. I have a lot to offer."

"Should I Live Moment by Moment or Make Plans for the Future?"

KATHLEEN

Kathleen, a PWA, lived with Jim. She, too, wanted to meet me before inviting me to their apartment. For the first interview, I talked with her at an agency, and the second interview took place in their kitchen. She described conflict about the right way to deal with the unpredictability of AIDS.

"I wasn't using drugs or doing things that are hazardous," Kathleen said. "But I trusted somebody. The person took a test and made sure it was negative. But the test was wrong. I was protective over getting AIDS, and I still got it. It's not fair to me. I can't make plans. I don't want to go to 5 years of college if I'm not going to live through it. I can't have kids."

"If I had more energy," she went on, "maybe I would have a better job and make more money, do something that I enjoyed. I don't have a car and those things people work 20 years for, and I don't think I'm going to get them. My life's got a time limit. I'm worried about dying. I'm young. My parents and everybody's going to outlive me. I love life, but I'm not going to be able to enjoy life like everybody else."

Describing her resolution to her conflict, she said, "I go day to day. I don't know how I'm going to feel, so I don't make plans. Most of my plans are going to the doctor or to school."

"I thought life was a big game," Kathleen reasoned. "Life is about peace, love, and happiness. Everybody should be taking care of everybody else because they're lucky that they're alive, and after you're dead, you don't exist anymore. Because of AIDS, I see what life is really about."

GREGG

Like Kathleen, Gregg described conflict about how he should deal with the unpredictability of AIDS. However, Gregg's experience was different from Kathleen's experience. Gregg said that he had AIDS and hemophilia, and since birth, he had experienced various chronic illnesses.

"I don't know how long I'll live," Gregg began. "Should I live for today or plan for the future? Can I justify the work, time, and money to go to college when I may not live to graduate? If I'm going to be dead soon, why study for a test when I could go to a concert? If I don't go to school, I don't know what to do with my time since I may have trouble getting and keeping a job because of AIDS. How can I come to grips with AIDS when I don't know what will happen next? I want to have a sense of control over my life."

"I decided to go to school," Gregg said about his resolution, "but I changed to a more satisfying major. Now I see my progress on a daily and weekly basis, and I don't feel as tense. I do what I can to come to grips with AIDS even though I don't know what will happen next. I try to have a positive attitude. I speak to groups about AIDS and read the transcripts of what I say so I get to know myself better. I participate in AIDS research."

Gregg rationalized, "Now my priority is happiness and personal satisfaction. It's important to enjoy what you do because you never know what's going to happen. I have become less materialistic than I was in high school when I wanted to get rich, have a big house and boat. To be happy, it's important to be, sit all alone and think. Because of the support of my friends and family, I don't feel alone."

"The more I come to grips with AIDS, the better my life is," Gregg continued. "People should always strive to make their life better. Why give up when I still have a chance? I don't have many other choices. I'm doing what I have to do to get by, to live. It isn't worth it to sit around and be bummed out. If I have only a year or two to be around, I don't want them to be a year or two of misery."

"Should I Continue to Use Expensive Treatment That Keeps Me Alive or Stop Using It and Die?"

NEAL

Neal, like Gregg, said that he had AIDS and hemophilia. He described conflict about the right way to deal with his guilt about his insurance company's expenditures on his health care. Without them, he would not receive treatment and would die.

"One surgery alone cost half a million dollars," Neal said. "I'm using health care at a rate several times what I'm paying. But I need health insurance to keep going and because I have a family. Getting health insurance is a tremendous concern if I ever look for another job."

Describing his resolution to his conflict, Neal said, "My big concern is self-preservation. To make up for what is being spent on me, I try to make a contribution. My family and I realized that the only way I was going to make my way and pay my keep was to get a good education. My education allows me to disappear when I'm ill and fulfill my job responsibilities by phone or proxy. I can be fairly sedentary."

"I have a life to live," Neal rationalized. "It would disturb me if I were not using my education for something. A good person will use the resources that were given. It's a responsibility for people to make a contribution. Intelligence and ability are God-given, and you shouldn't hide it but use it."

"Should I Take Dope (Prescribed Medication) to Control My Pain Even Though It Isn't Good for Me?"

BUD

Bud, a PWA, had a history of homelessness and drug abuse, but because of various chronic illnesses, he had agreed to live in an inner-city apartment. He described conflict about the right way to control his pain.

"My whole body hurts just about all the time," said Bud. "I don't eat that good because I can't stand up long enough to fix it. Now the pain got so bad I have to use pills. It's really dope. They help me. The pain stopped for a while. Then started back, and I have to get more dope. I almost died twice since I've been taking that heavy stuff by taking too much with constant pains. I don't like to take dope because I don't want to put them in my body. When I took that methadone, and the pain went away, it felt so good to sit down and not hurt anymore. Only the dope is strong enough to take away my pain."

"Now I stay home and drink beer and pop pills," Bud said concerning his resolution to his conflict. "I read the paper, sleep in my chair, go to sleep. I take methadone 7 days a week. I got three a day to take, but if one do the job I don't have to take three."

Bud reasoned, "I stay home because I have too much pain to wait for a bus or go anyplace. I only take as much methadone as I need, as long as the methadone helps the pain. I'd rather not take more than one if I don't have to. I'm not taking them to get high. If I wanted to get high I wouldn't mess with that no way. I'd go on the streets and get my drugs. See, I like street drugs is how I do drugs."

"How Should I Balance the Needs of My Children, My Loved One With AIDS, and Myself?"

CAROLYN

Carolyn, a significant person, walked into the living room after her boyfriend, a PWA, completed his interview and left for work. During her interview, Carolyn described conflict about the right way to balance the needs of her children, her boyfriend, and herself.

"How would I do this?" she asked. "It mean I have to do the driving, more doctors' appointments, taking care of his needs plus my sons' and mine. All of that would not get done. Don't too much get done now."

In resolution to her conflict, Carolyn explained, "I've been to the doctor. I've learned how to do his shots. If he ever got sick, I could do the things that he's been doing. So it wasn't like turning my back on him. I do all the doctor calling and making different appointments. I'm being like a mother to him and a girlfriend. It's like I'm one person with two brains. I have to work for me and my kids and plus for him. When I feel like I need time out, he does give it to me."

Carolyn rationalized, "I'm sure one day there will be a cure for AIDS. Then again, there may not. You don't get it from drinking and casual contact or anything because if that was true I would have had it by now. My mom has her disability. I was used to taking care of her and my two little sisters. I'm still taking care of a household. But it's not as much as with my mom. The main step is getting involved and making them feel like nothing's really wrong with them."

Commentary

The eight PWAs who described ethical problems involving AIDS as a chronic illness talked about their frustration with their deteriorating health, the unpredictability of their lives, the cost of their health care, and their pain. As Matthew said, "It's scary to be young and have a disease that can take over." Under these circumstances, they questioned the right way to live.

Trying to adjust to their deteriorating health, the PWAs said they wanted to live as fully and as long as possible under the circumstances. "Why give up when I still have a chance?" Gregg asked. "I don't have many other choices." Jim said, "Life is worth living. By making changes, I want to put off death because I don't feel like I've accomplished anything." Mary explained in words that were repeated by all 25 PWAs, "You have to accept [AIDS] and go on with your life. Life is precious."

The PWAs' stories illustrate many of the difficulties involved with managing life while experiencing a chronic, life-threatening illness. PWAs and their loved ones must cope with opportunistic infections that produce major changes in their life-styles and arrange their lives around inevitable crises regarding their health. Symptom control becomes a paramount issue (Ragsdale, Kotarba, & Morrow, 1992).

Because of the increasing number of persons with chronic illness, society has been grappling with ethical problems regarding the right way to address their health care needs in ways that are humane and cost-effective (Benjamin, 1988; Beresford, 1989; Cockerell & Nary, 1991; Davis, 1991; Fox, 1990; Fuerst, 1991; Hutman, 1991). Health care resources are costly and limited. Many PWAs, such as

Bud, do not have insurance or are underinsured (Lewis, 1989; Moseley, 1989). Even PWAs, like Neal, who can afford private health insurance must rely on other people to help fund their health care.

The dominant goal of the health care system has been to cure people and fully restore their functioning by using high technology. Some ethicists have argued that this goal may not be appropriate for treating persons with chronic illness (Jennings, Callahan, & Caplan, 1988). Questions arise about when high technology is appropriate therapy. Neal received an expensive hip replacement as a palliative treatment. Should high technology be used for palliation when cure is not possible? If not, what are the alternatives (Durham, 1991; Fins, 1992)?

The focus of treatment for PWAs is rightfully shifting from acute, inpatient care of terminally ill persons to outpatient, long-term care. Obstacles to outpatient care include a shortage of workers who are trained and willing to provide PWAs with home care (Cassidy, 1991) and resistance among staff and residents of long-term care facilities to admission of PWAs. Education programs and cost projection studies may help to alleviate some of these problems (Allers, 1990; Gwartney, Daly, Roccaforte, & Smith, 1992). Experience with other chronically ill individuals can guide the development of humane, cost-effective, and equitable health care services for PWAs (Benjamin, 1989; Oppenheimer & Padgug, 1991).

Ideally, a multidisciplinary continuum of services would be offered to PWAs and other chronically ill persons. These services would unify often inflexible and disparate segments of the health care system into a more adaptable, coordinated whole. They would include home care, long-term care, day care, respite care, supported housing, hospice care, and acute care. This care would be tailored to meet the specific needs of women, lesbians and gay men, and people of color (Bilheimer, Asher, Phillips, & Smith, 1991; Fahs et al., 1992; Levine, 1990b; Moore, 1991).

The PWAs and significant persons talked about what they themselves were doing to resolve their ethical problems involving chronic illness. Their experience may benefit anyone who is confronted by ethical problems involving chronic illness. Support from friends, family, health care workers, and society would enhance the success of such activities (Ragsdale et al., 1992; Ragsdale & Morrow, 1990).

Not all of the participants' experiences were negative. They also discussed how AIDS was affecting their values in a positive manner. As Kathleen put it, "Life is about peace, love, and happiness. Everybody should be taking care of everybody else because they're lucky that they're alive. Because of AIDS, I see what life is really about." Jackie explained, "You can make life good and happy, in spite of everything. To be able to enjoy what you can, give what you can give. Because the opposite kind of life isn't worth living."

In summary, society has responsibility to address the health care needs of PWAs and other individuals with chronic illness in ways that are humane and cost-effective. Learning from the participants' example, persons with chronic illness can do their part by staying alive, living as "normally" as possible, taking good care of themselves, reaching out for help, concentrating on the present, and contributing to society. Their loved ones can utilize community resources to learn about and adapt to the chronic illness. By working together, society and individuals will be able to develop resolutions that lead to meaning and integrity.

6

Ethical Problems Involving Death

Human beings long to escape death and achieve eternal life. In order to avoid being reminded of their mortality, people often inadvertently shun, isolate, and discount dying persons. The social stigma can also extend to individuals who are bereaved because of their association with someone who is dying (Jonas, 1992). AIDS heightens people's fears about death. In examining the metaphors of AIDS, Sontag (1989) wrote that society views AIDS like an invading enemy, linking AIDS and death, and blames PWAs. Friends, family, clergy, health care personnel, and PWAs themselves connect AIDS and death (Flanagan, 1990; Lo, 1989).

The participants talked more about death than any other topic. Consequently, this chapter is longer than other chapters about the content of their ethical problems. At the time that I conducted the research, AIDS was considered to be fatal, although the life span and quality of life of persons with HIV disease were increasing (Levine, 1990b). The participants indicated that they were aware of the connection between AIDS and death, although they hoped that they or their loved one with AIDS would be able to beat the odds. They described what they were doing to avoid or come to terms with their mortality.

Nine PWAs (five women and four men) and three significant persons (one woman and two men) specifically described ethical problems involving death: "Should I give in to my fears about death or view death from a spiritual perspective?" "Should I live the way that I feel like living or live in a way that will assure me of going to heaven when I die?" "Should I commit suicide, which may be wrong?" "Should I write a living will even though I don't want to think about my death?" "How should I live fully while helping my loved one to experience a good death?"

"Should I Give In to My Fears About Death or View Death From a Spiritual Perspective?"

CLAUDIA

I interviewed Claudia, a PWA, in the hospital because she wanted to talk with me right away in case she died before being discharged. Several days later, Claudia, in fact, went home, where I met her for her second interview. During her first interview, she lay in her hospital bed and described conflict about whether she should give in to her fears about death or view death from a spiritual perspective.

"I've been in shock since that man from the health department told me I had HIV and I'm going to die," Claudia said. "My health is gone downhill. I throw up everything. All of a sudden, you're getting blood transfusions, and your fingers and feet are swelling, and you're taking medicine, and it's supposed to be helping, but it don't. It's scary because it's all new to you. Nobody thinks they're going to die young. Everybody thinks they're going to live till they catch some old people's disease. Dying is scary because I'm too young. I got kids."

Although Claudia said that she had not resolved her conflict, she was taking action to come to terms with her diagnosis. "Everything that comes on TV," she said, "I sit with my eyes glued because I want to learn more about my disease. I want to hear if they have a cure. When they have the story of the [Names Project] quilt on, I recorded that because I thought that was some good information for people to know."

Claudia reasoned, "Everybody ignores AIDS until you get it. You can pass it on so quickly. Sharing needles is a no-no. God, it's scary. You will die. You got to make plans right away because you

never know when you're going to keel over. When you die, you
leave the earth. Your body's still there but your insides aren't. You
can't have fun any more. You can't take your kids to the movies
or buy your kids nothing."

CHRIS

Before his interview, Chris, a PWA, showed me his family pho-
tographs, saying that he wanted me to know how he used to look.
I saw images of a young athlete that contrasted sharply with his
present, emaciated appearance. He noticed my tears and smiled
at me with the same warmth that I saw in his eyes in the photo-
graphs. Then, we sat down at the kitchen table and he described
conflict about whether he should give in to his fears about death
or view death from a spiritual perspective.

"My aunt died when I was 6," Chris said, "and I wasn't afraid
to see her lying dead on the couch. I loved her. My mother gave
me straight answers about her, and that demystified death. Even
though I learned that death is change, which is part of life and
natural, change can be threatening because it makes you feel
vulnerable."

Describing his resolution to his conflict, Chris said, "Since being
diagnosed with AIDS, I've experienced many changes, and I've
learned to accept them. Materialism and greed keep us from
experiencing fully the wonders of life. Now materialism doesn't
control my life like it did before. I focus on the present instead of
the future. The present is the most wonderful experience I've ever
had. I have a wonderful warm feeling for the past."

"I am dying, but so is everyone else," rationalized Chris. "I feel
the loving presence of my uncle. When I've walked through that
doorway, the same feeling will be present with people who love
me. We can choose what's on the other side of the door."

"I feel close to people who have confronted their mortality,"
Chris continued. "We share the secret that we have nothing to fear
from death. Through interaction, sharing, warmth, and love that
little secret grows and is supportive. By believing the secret, I am
more centered and focused on love, life, and those emotions that

make us the wonderful spiritual beings that we are. Death is part of life, not the end of life. I'm a hundred percent sure there is something beyond death. The wonderful part is not knowing what comes after death."

RUTH

Ruth, a PWA, was a large, strong-looking woman whose presence seemed to fill her living room where I sat talking with her young children while she got ready for my interview with her. When we were alone, I was surprised that she, like Claudia and Chris, described conflict about whether to give in to her fears about death or view death from a spiritual perspective.

"I'm scared of death," Ruth said. "I don't want to die. I don't want to leave my children early. When I found out about having AIDS, I was devastated, maybe because I was told that I was going to die. So I came home and went to bed to die. After 3 days, my friend put me in her bed where I stayed 3 more days. I prayed and drifted off to sleep. I dreamed I was picking cotton. It was a whole field of cotton all budded, beautiful, and white, and I knew then that I wasn't going to die because the field was not finished. I says, 'I'm hungry,' and I got out of bed. That was the beginning of a new start for me."

"I can't give up," Ruth said about her resolution. "Even when I'm not feeling well, I push me. It doesn't come easy. I don't focus on AIDS. Now I'm living in Christ. I'm not as afraid to die as I was. I don't want to leave my kids. I love them. But I'm going to get peace about them."

"I got so much to live for—me, my kids," Ruth said, explaining her rationale. "I have life in me, and I'm going to hope till I can't breath anymore. Not to be cured of HIV, because I am cured, and to be cured is to go on. I look at my children, and it's like a injection. There's somebody else that need to know that you don't have to give up. If I focused on AIDS, I'd probably commit suicide. One day, I almost got killed by a car because I didn't see a light turn red. That was a miracle, and I began to learn how to live."

"My hope is in God," said Ruth. "Everything that I did wrong, He forgave me, and I'm blessed. I was on my knees praying, and

I was scared to die. This voice said, 'You're already dead in me, but yet you live.' I began to know that it was the power of God that was keeping me."

"I don't have that terrible fear of death anymore," Ruth continued. "Something about death give me a sweetness, when I know it's going to be all right. I had a dream about a guy who died of AIDS. He said to me, 'Don't worry about death. It's sweet.' He say, 'I'm OK,' and he looked so good, so rested. Inside me, it's a laughter. I can't describe it, I don't know how it happened, but it's there. It's a juiciness, a sugarness. Death was a big issue but not anymore."

"Should I Live the Way That I Feel Like Living or in a Way That Will Assure Me of Going to Heaven When I Die?"

ROBERT

Robert, a PWA, talked about death, just as Claudia, Chris, and Ruth did. However, he described conflict about whether to live the way that he felt like living or in a way that would assure him of going to heaven when he died.

"If they tell you that you're going to die," Robert said, "that's a shock for a guy who thought he was going to live until he's 60. It was scary to think that I wouldn't exist. I wondered what was the right way to have a good life on earth and then go to heaven when I die? If there isn't life after death, why try in this life? Should my belief about eternal life affect how I live my life?"

Robert described his resolution to his conflict. "The biggest thing that I have accomplished is learning to live with death," he said. "I put my trust in God, and I'm not as afraid of dying. I'm more at peace than I've ever been in my life. I've accepted that I'm going to die, and so is everybody else."

"When I was diagnosed with AIDS," Robert said, explaining his rationale, "I didn't care if I lived or died. I was alone in the hospital and losing hope. Hope means feeling that life is worth living. A nurse sat by me, held my hand, and encouraged me. She told me,

'There's more to life. Keep going, keep fighting, and it will work out.' Without her, I don't know if I would have made it. She made me feel great. I went back and thanked her after I was well and looked good again. On a regular basis, I stop by the hospital floors that I've been on and talk to them and tell them how good I'm doing."

"I was visited by the Holy Spirit," Robert continued. "My brother took me to a spiritual retreat. He grabbed the minister and said, 'Would you pray over my brother who's got AIDS?' We sat in chairs and made a circle. The man put his hand on me and started praying. My legs shaked, my arms shaked, my head shaked. Since then my attitude has changed."

"God is in everything and we are his children," Robert said. "Believing in life after death takes away some of the fear of death and affects how I live. I have zeal for life because I want to help people. I'm trying to be a good person, doing what is right. If there is a heaven, I'll go there after I die. The right way to live is to treat everybody fair. Don't offend God, other people, yourself. Don't steal. Don't tell a lie."

"If you're a good person, you alleviate sin, doing what's wrong," Robert said. "You instinctively know if you do something wrong. If you ask forgiveness from God and the person you offended and do your best to keep from sinning, your slate is wiped clean, if you truly mean it. You feel better about life, and you will be rewarded in eternal life. If I didn't have God to trust in, I'd have a difficult time."

RALPH

Ralph, a PWA, looked weak and sickly. I wanted to put my arms around him and give him strength. Like Robert, he described conflict about whether he should live in the way that he felt like living or in a way that would assure him of going to heaven when he died. With only a fourth grade education, he contrasted sharply with Robert, a college graduate.

"Am I going to die from AIDS?" Ralph asked. "I don't have any people I can talk with about this. I was in Vegas when I got sick. I sits in the hospital and read about different dudes that had AIDS. I be wondering, is this going to happen to me? I was sleeping in a room with a Black dude. Man, he looked bad. I was thinking, I'm going to be like that?"

"Hey man," Ralph went on, "that don't bother me about dying. Then I thinking about how to get straight with God. Only thing I thought would help me was God. I'm talking about my soul. If I die, I will go to heaven if I straighten things out with God. Otherwise I'll go to hell."

Describing his resolution to his conflict, Ralph said, "God and I have a private discussion. I think that's who I be talking to. I talk to him just like me and you talk. Get on my knees, if I could get up. If I can't get up, I lay there and talk to him. I tell him to forgive me for all bad things. Every time I get in trouble, I run to God and promise him this and that. He knows I'm not telling the truth. That kind of bother me. I'm tired of lying to Him. I be meaning to straighten things out with God, but haven't done it yet."

"I go to God," Ralph reasoned, "and I ain't got nothing to worry about. He have hope for me. God helps me every day I wake up and find out that I'm still alive. I know a lot of people praying for me. That helps me feel better. I haven't straightened things out with God, but he still bless me. I always talked to God. I always believed in God. Dying is easy, living is the hard part."

MARGARET

I interviewed Margaret, a PWA, in her inner-city apartment. We sat down on the couch, and she reached out to clasp my hand, which she held firmly throughout the interview. Like Robert and Ralph, she described conflict about whether she should live in the way that she felt like living or in a way that would assure her of going to heaven when she died.

"There's so many people living bad lives, why did God pick me to get AIDS?" Margaret asked. "How do I make peace with God so I'm not afraid of dying, and I'll go to heaven? A lot of people are afraid of dying because they don't know where they're going after death. They believe they be punished in hell because of what they did. It's frightening to be separated from God, but it's a tremendous thing to know where you're going."

"I've made peace with God and other people," Margaret said about her resolution to her conflict. "I am trying to live a clean, right life so I have a good death and go to heaven. You have to change your whole life-style. That's what God wants you to do. I'm not afraid of dying because I know that I'm going to heaven. I'll be out of my pain."

Describing her rationale, Margaret said, "If you're at peace with other people and God, you can have a peaceful death and go to heaven. You wouldn't be scared of anything. You wouldn't leave this life with hurt people and guilt. That's bad for you. The right way to live is to try not to sin. You'll have more quality of life. You know in your heart what God's rules are. When you break them, God's going to give you a chance to redeem yourself. One needs forgiveness to have inner peace, and then your actions show it."

"Should I Commit Suicide, Which May be Wrong?"

JACK

Jack said that he did not want anyone, other than his wife, his nurse, and his physician, to know that he had AIDS. To protect his confidentiality, we met secretly in my office early on a Saturday morning. Jack, who had a Ph.D., described conflict about whether to commit suicide.

"It's the uncertainty that gets you," Jack said. "I don't know how long I will live or what will happen to me after I die. My supreme fear has been a loss of mental faculties. Surviving may be worse than black nothingness, if that's what's next. You may get into a syndrome where you have lost all health coverage, and you don't want to be a burden on the family. In those circumstances, I wonder if I would commit suicide."

Describing his resolution to his conflict, Jack said, "I treat the uncertainty about death as something that I have to make accommodations for and go on. It's made me stronger in faith. During this last bout with pneumonia, I was on full respirator. When I lived, I became a Roman Catholic. I have made my family my priority over work."

"Right now," Jack continued, "I'm not giving up, and suicide is a form of giving up. If I were to commit suicide, I would not choose anything lingering. I would do it in consultation with my wife, if I'm competent. I probably wouldn't do it unless she would be in agreement. I wouldn't want her to be affected by the stigma at church."

Jack reasoned, "My life is too pleasurable to commit suicide at this time. God may not guide me to commit suicide, but God would forgive me, which is a loophole. I can't condemn somebody who commits suicide because I'm not in their shoes. What keeps me from committing suicide is my belief that there's something I've gotta do, so it's not time to die yet. I should have died and haven't. Something had to intervene so I would survive."

"My view about life after death is a change in state," said Jack. "Hell is the absence of heaven, if there is a heaven, not devils and fire. My beliefs about death don't influence how I live my life now. If you go with the morals that you were raised with, you don't have to worry about the penalties after death."

SALLY

Like Jack, Sally, a PWA, described conflict about whether to commit suicide. However, their perspectives differed. Jack, who previously had engaged in postdoctoral study, held an upper middle-class professional position. Sally, who had dropped out of school after the sixth grade, said that she was "on welfare."

"Should I overdose on cocaine?" Sally asked. "I may be in constant pain, skinny, losing my hair. And people got to take care of me. And I can't go to the bathroom by myself, can't dress myself, can't feed myself. It's miserable because of HIV. You can't plan ahead. That pisses me off because when I have something that I want to do with my children, something gets in the way. God, when is this going to end? I'm scared about what will happen to me."

"I probably would commit suicide if my husband would go before me," Sally continued. "He said I wasn't satisfied, when he told me he had HIV, until I had HIV. I was going to do what I could do to get it, and I don't understand that. I guess because I don't want to lose him. If something did happen, I want it to happen to me before him. I couldn't take it. If I didn't have my kids, I probably wouldn't live. I feel like I'm living for my children, not myself."

"The biggest fear is fear of death," she said. "I don't believe there is anything after death. It's probably wrong to say. They say, 'I'm going to heaven. I want to see you there.' Oh Jesus, it's tiresome hearing [that] all the time. Not existing is frightening. Sometimes I get scared to go to bed because I don't know if I'm going to wake up and that's going to be an end."

Sally described her resolution. "If I have a short time to live," she said, "I'm going to take an overdose of cocaine. I don't want people to take care of me. I want my kids to see me like they remember me before I did get this disease. I try to take care of myself as best I can to prolong my life."

Explaining her rationale for her resolution, Sally said, "I don't want to live and die in pain. I want to die right away. I want to live as long as possible because I want to see my kids grow up, get married, and have kids. I want to see their kids grow up. If I die I miss out on all of that."

"Should I Write a Living Will Even Though I Don't Want to Think About My Death?"

KIMBERLY

Kimberly, a PWA, told me that previously she had injected drugs. In order to maintain her sobriety, she was trying to straighten out her life. For her, that included preparing for her death, even though she did not want to think about death. She described conflict about whether to make out a living will.

"I don't want to be kept alive by life support," Kimberly said. "I want to have control. My family would probably keep me alive with a bunch of crap. When I'm supposed to die naturally, I want to go. This doesn't mean that I'm not going to do things to prevent that. I should write a living will, but I haven't because it makes me look at my mortality more. I've had the paperwork for a year. I should also make out a will, but a living will is most important."

"Right now," she resolved, "I'm doing nothing about the living will. It's sitting in my file cabinet. It's a matter of pushing myself because I don't want to look at the end result. I've come half-way around, but I haven't gone full circle." Explaining her rationale for her resolution, Kimberly said, "It's scary to think about death even though I've accepted it. People don't want to talk about death because we want to live. Death is nonexistence, which is frightening. AIDS has made me want to live. It's been positive in turning my life around, helping me quit drugs. I've met wonderful people. I don't spend time with people I'm iffy about. I have new activities. I have some self-respect. Knowing that my time is shortened, I've wanted to change the quality of it."

"How Should I Live Fully While Helping My Loved One to Experience a Good Death?"

PETER

Peter, a significant person, was the first participant to use the term *good death*. Initially, I thought this term was a contradiction. "How can death from AIDS be good?" I asked myself. However, the more that I listened to Peter and the other participants, the more they taught me about a good death. Peter described conflict about how to live his own life fully while helping his lover to experience a good death.

"Should I take care of him even though he won't be alive to take care of me when I become ill?" Peter asked. "He might die slowly. It could be horrible. I want to be with him during his death, but I also want to leave him and find someone else so that I won't be alone. It's painful. What kind of a person should I be so that I can go on living after he dies? How should I balance my needs with his needs? How should I live my life so that I have a good death myself?"

"I will take care of him and develop a support system to help out," resolved Peter. "I'm giving him more love because our time together may be limited. I don't want to hurt him. I want to be with him when he dies so he won't die alone. I am trying to be a good person so I can feel good about myself after he dies. I give greater value to intimacy, love, trust, relationships, life. I try to be more understanding of other people's feelings."

Peter explained his rationale by saying, "I love him, and he deserves to be treated well. We need to be as supportive and caring of each other as we can, especially if time is limited. Being a good person is right for me. Right means what is my nature, what's comfortable for me. It fits me. This doesn't mean it's right for someone else. It comes from inside of me and isn't imposed from the outside."

JAMES

James, a significant person, and I met in my office because his lover's parents were visiting, and he did not want them to know about our conversation. His eyes filled with tears as he described conflict about how he should live fully while helping his lover to experience a good death.

"Should I help him commit suicide?" James asked. "I want him to live, but not if he doesn't want to. I'm afraid he might commit suicide, and I'll find him dead. If he does, I hope he leaves me a letter that says that he loves me. He might commit suicide because of dementia and blindness, but I don't think so. You come to the point where you have it, and you find out you can live with it. It's hard to say what would make him decide to let go. It would be, it's time to go, I've worked hard enough, I need to rest."

"Dealing with his death is so painful that it lowers my self-esteem," James said. "If he dies, not only will I lose him, but my dreams. I may lose our house, his family, our friends. I feel more susceptible to hurt, and I hesitate showing this vulnerability to other people. I withhold myself from other people in order to protect myself, and my self-esteem suffers."

Describing his resolution to his conflict, James said, "I encourage him to talk openly and honestly about dying, to embrace death, without giving up. I am trying to take things one day at a time. We are beginning to plan his funeral so things go the way he wants, and I can cry. I spend time with people who are supportive, loving, caring. As far as helping him to commit suicide, I will err on the side of life. We have been talking with his parents about how he wants to die. We will discuss his death with his doctor and take care of the legal problems."

James rationalized, "I want to help him die with peace, not anger. To have a sense that he's done everything he needs to. That he accepts dying. I want to help him have a sense of God or higher power. I will feel better about his death if he's peaceful." Blowing his nose, James said, "My tears are about surviving. It's frightening to think that I'm going to be alone. I've never been in as much love with anybody."

"I want to be with him when he dies," said James, "because I think I would be comforting for him, and I love him. That I could help him. I want to say to him, 'You can go. I can carry on. I want you to be happy.' I want him to know he's loved and comforted into his death."

MEAGAN

Meagan, a significant person, met me in my office so that her roommate would not know about our conversation. A graduate student, she described conflict about how to live fully herself while helping her boyfriend to experience a good death.

"At night," Meagan began, "I worry about his possible death. What if I am waiting for him, and he doesn't come because he is dead? What if he commits suicide? If he would die, it would affect school, work, friends, myself, future relationships, parents, shopping, everything. I don't know how to handle my grief about what we would have together if he lived a long life."

Describing her resolution, Meagan said, "I try to be optimistic but also deal realistically with AIDS. I try to control my worrying about his possible death. I try to find ways that I can help out. I can't do anything medically, but I can help him psychologically by keeping his spirits up."

Meagan explained her rationale. "I would rather be in control than not," she said. "I don't like to think that there is nothing I can do to help him. If he was depressed all the time, he would be more susceptible to illness. When I encourage him, he is more open to things he should be doing, like taking medications."

Experience of a "Good Death"

The previous sections consist of the participants' ethical problems that they described during their initial interviews. Several participants contributed more to the research than their initial interviews. Kirsten and Tony, Carlos, Jeffrey and Sonia, and Mark and Nick shared their experience of a good death.

KIRSTEN AND TONY

In her audiotaped validation interview, Kirsten, a PWA, described conflict about how to experience a good death. A registered nurse, she said that she valued feeling good about dying, but she also valued taking care of her husband, Tony.

"I'm sad about leaving him," Kirsten said. "He'll have a hard time coping with the basics of life. He'll be lonely and unhappy." She stopped to blow her nose. "My tears are because I don't want him to be unhappy. I wish he didn't have to go through this because of me. We should try to resolve this because it's not resolved now. We've talked a little and kidded about it. I wouldn't mind if he finds somebody else and gets married. That would give him a happier life."

Tony's eyes filled with tears during his second interview as he described conflict about how to help Kirsten experience a good death. "After the first interview," he said, "we began to talk about how she can have a good death. A person wants a loved one not to suffer and to go peacefully. I read articles on letting go. A person lies in bed, struggling. Finally, there is a turning point. The dying person lets go. The loved ones let go, too. Nurses and doctors are trained to make people well, but they aren't trained to help people face up to death."

After Kirsten died, Tony sent me a letter saying that her death had been "good." He gave permission for the letter to be part of the research. "She had asked me to help her go home with dignity and without long suffering," Tony wrote, "and I promised I would do my best to carry out her wishes. I would vacillate from acceptance of the situation to a far-away hope that she would somehow come back to normal, and I would be able to take her home. Then, I am sure under the hand of God, other events helped me face reality—events such as her direct request to the doctor, 'Doctor, this isn't living—you must help me.' "

"I feel satisfied and sad/happy for the way everything happened at her passing. She very much preferred to breathe her last in the hospital with us by her side. I think even in this she was thinking of me so I wouldn't have memories of her dying in our own bed. The AIDS virus allows one a great deal of time for personal togetherness—and we made good use of our time.

"Her courage and faith included a large portion of love and strength that she gave to me to enable me to help her throughout her illness and, perhaps more importantly, to enable me to help her at the time of her journey home. With her love and her help, I have only feelings of contentment and satisfaction, with no regrets— and I am sure she smiles down on all of us today. Her courage and her faith are now her lasting gift to all of us."

CARLOS

Over a 3-month period, Carlos, a PWA, wrote five letters describing his thoughts about a good death. I assume that he died when the letters stopped. This section contains portions of these letters in the order in which he sent them to me.

"No drug is as powerful as hope. You can't overdose on it, and it's free for everyone. If hope fades, maybe we are relying too much on ourselves, or we need to have faith that we are protected and loved by other people and God. I try to spread hope. I don't see or hear as well as I did, I could be impotent, and I have abominable infirmities, but nothing destroys my hope."

"There are many paths to a fulfilling spiritual life. Few people walk the same pathway, though they may walk in the same direction. We know when we are on the right path because it is paved with love. Because of God and other people, the path is not lonely. We must be true to our highest self, despite difficulty, for this is the path."

"Death can seem abrupt, but love heals grief. I've had so much grief in my 40 years that I feel twice my age. Love gives me strength, understanding, and emotional release that makes room for reassurance and oneness. The extremes of human experience bring me deeper into the love of God and unity with others both here and beyond—for love never ends!"

"Hell doesn't come after death. We will experience love unending and reunion. When my time arrives, I will know the Gatekeeper by name. I am excited at the prospects that await me after this life. I am anxious to know what is now the unknowable, to see the unseeable, to experience the impossible to experience."

"I have been having awful dreams in which I am trying to fix my childhood, that is just out of reach. I awake crying. My analyst said I am not much different from other adults with a history of child abuse. But since my life span is limited, my unconscious self is working overtime to make peace with my past. Many people living with AIDS have to face their demons younger and less prepared than their predecessors. Some of us rise to the occasion but others pass over to the other side carrying that luggage. I find this most unappetizing."

"Forgiven and forgiving, nurtured, loved, and at peace with the Creator, death comes even so. Why? I don't know. I am certain that God is greater than AIDS. I shall not get to choose how I will die, or when. But I can decide how I am going to live. Life is about choices."

"Last week paramedics took me to the hospital. I saw my dearest friends crying and hovering over me. Time went by like a series of snapshots, poorly posed, with dark shadows dodging nurses, doctors, technicians. The colors seemed pea green, warm, interspersed with white jackets. I woke to see my mother's face, eyes swollen and red from crying, her hands desperately clutching mine, saying, 'Don't go.' My father stood behind her with furrowed brow, ashen face. I rallied. With so much love holding me back, why go now? Stay. Fight the good fight. Any moment, science will find a cure for AIDS."

"My parents went back this morning. It was terrible saying goodbye. They wanted to take me home with them, but I insisted on my own life and death. I cannot fathom my mother's sorrow; perhaps that's what holds me back. I am becoming more focused on what I can do to ease them into quiet acceptance. This is part of their growth. I make it a point to bring laughter into our conversations and to matter-of-factly deal with mortality—nobody gets out of here alive."

"Dying is meant to be a shared experience. It takes uncommon courage to be with someone who is dying, to say goodbye, and rejoice through sadness. The decision to let the person live on through you perpetuates the dignity of his or her life and validates your highest self. A part of you goes with the person. A part of the person remains forever in you. As caregiver, nurturer, healer in the difficult places of the heart, you step closer to the truth."

"I am becoming preoccupied with death, but not morosely. The transition to nonmortal being comes easier and more naturally than I first supposed. I feel anticipation. My only fear is that death will come at the hands of violence, will harm my survivors, or will be drawn out and painful."

"I will pursue my career and get well. I refuse to give up. Sunrise and sunset are beautiful in my eyes for I seek to see through the eyes of the Creator. Everyone is expecting me to pull off another miracle. Would I let them down? Of course not. Not any more than I would let myself down."

"This week I feel better. I am going to the fair to look at pigs and eat corn on the cob cooked over a mesquite fire and dripping with butter. I like to buy mango chutney, peach preserves, and jalapeno sweet pickles to be served as side dishes with beef ribs, new potatoes, cornbread, and a colorful, chunky green salad. I will get up, dust myself off, and get back on track. Besides, I have to wait around to read your dissertation. Wouldn't miss that for nuthin'!"

JEFFREY AND SONIA

The day after Jeffrey died from AIDS, Sonia, his mother, called me to say that he wanted his death to be part of the research. She explained that his death was "good" because her ethical problem ("Although I value the expertise of my son's doctor, should I get another doctor who has a heart?") was effectively resolved. Sonia said that she obtained Jeffrey's release from prison so that he could go home to die, and she quit her job to take care of him. During that time, they said what they wanted to say to each other. He asked to be cremated and have her scatter some of his ashes over his beloved ocean and forest and keep the rest at home so that she could talk to them.

A week before dying, Jeffrey was hospitalized. Because his regular physician was not available, Jeffrey was assigned to a physician who, Sonia said, "cradled my heart." This physician comforted her by holding her hand and treating Jeffrey respectfully. He had a cot put in Jeffrey's room so that Sonia could stay overnight. All week, he visited them regularly, and he told them that they were special. He could not do much for Jeffrey, but because he nurtured Sonia, she was able to nurture her son. She said that God brought him for Jeffrey's last week.

Sonia and the physician made the decision not to put Jeffrey on life support. "Why prolong the inevitable?" she asked. She said that she and Jeffrey were not afraid. Because they were at peace, she gave him permission to die, and he gave her permission to go on with her life.

Since Jeffrey was lying peacefully, Sonia went to brush her teeth. He waited for her so that she would be there when he died. When she came back, his breathing became less and less, and it finally stopped. He died as "I cradled him in my arms." His death was "peaceful and good, nothing to fear."

Sonia cried as she described the loss of her son. To be close to him, she sat in his room where she felt his presence. She listened to his music, and she talked to him. She said that she could see him smiling and riding bareback in the wind, feeling free and peaceful.

MARK AND NICK

During their initial interviews, Mark, a PWA, and Nick, his lover, described conflict about what they should do so that Mark would experience a good death and Nick "would be able to go on living afterward." Several months later, Nick asked me to conduct a third audiotaped interview of Mark, to be used as the basis of Mark's memorial service and a letter to his family. Mark donated the interview to the research.

As Mark invited me into his living room, I felt sad to see how much his health had deteriorated since my second interview with him. However, he gave me a warm hug as he had done previously. After turning on the tape recorder, I tried to think of questions that Mark's loved ones would want to ask him after he died. "How do you want to be remembered?" I asked.

"I hope they remember me as somebody who made their life a little better," he said. "That they smile and laugh when they think of me. I'd like them to remember the good side of things."

"What are you most proud of about your life?" I asked.

"That I have not intentionally caused harm," he said. "I was blind in one eye and progressively blind in the other. I decided that I could not take the risk of killing anyone, so I stopped driving. It was a hard decision because of giving up my power."

"What values are important to you?" I asked.

"My values changed after I was diagnosed with AIDS," he said. "The emphasis in society is on materialism. I'm not proud of working for money even though it has given me insurance and other benefits. I've had time to think about things. What is important to me now is being able to give love. If you give love, you get love."

"Do you have any regrets about your life?" I asked.

"Not about being gay," he said. "I regret that AIDS is putting a quicker end to my life than I would like. If I had it to do again, I would like to give more to society than paperwork and making money. I didn't think about that until it was too late. I've helped people, but I could have done more."

"What do you believe about God?" I asked.

"I believe in God," he said, "but I don't believe in organized religion because too often it involves bad things, like hate of homosexuality. There is nothing wrong with homosexuality. AIDS is a virus, not a judgment of God. God wouldn't make AIDS to punish people."

"What do you believe about death?" I asked.

"I believe there's life after death but I don't know what it is like," Mark said. "Sometimes I look forward to death because I'm curious. I'm convinced that death will be good. I plan to be cremated. At my memorial service, I want the people who are there to feel my love and I want to feel their love. That would be satisfying for my soul."

"What kind of death would you like to have, so you have a good death?" I asked.

"I would like to be at home with Nick and my mother and father," he said. "They would hold my hands and give me permission to go on. I have a living will signed. They understand why I don't want to go on indefinitely. I don't want to be in a state where I'm not consciously aware of anything or I can't communicate decently with other people."

Two days later, I delivered the audiotape and printout of the interview to Mark's house. A month later, Nick asked if I could come and say goodbye to Mark. Nick said that Mark had decided to stop all medications and die at home rather than in a hospital, just as he had described in his third interview. The next day after talking with Nick and Mark's parents, I walked upstairs to Mark's bedroom where he was lying in bed covered with a yellow quilt. Flowers, books, music, and a bird cage filled the room. I kissed him on the forehead, sat down by him, and held his hand. He did not say anything, but he squeezed my hand.

"I will never forget you," I said, trying to think of what would comfort him. "Thank you for contributing to the research. I admire you because you've courageously faced life and death. You are showing me how to experience a good death. Nick and your parents will miss you because no one will take your place, but I think they will be fine. Your body is tired. It's all right if you want to go on. It won't be scary. You will feel more peace, joy, and love than you've ever felt before." After sitting by him for awhile and talking quietly, I told him that I was leaving. I kissed him again, and he squeezed my hand again.

Downstairs, I was putting on my coat when Mark's mother said that his breathing had changed. Concerned about Mark feeling pain, she called the doctor, who said that a nurse would be there in an hour to begin an intravenous infusion and administer morphine. Mark's parents and Nick had read the transcript of Mark's third interview in which he had said that he wanted to die naturally at home. They were committed to helping Mark to die as he wanted. But now, confronted with the reality of Mark's death, they seemed frightened. They said that they had never seen anyone die at home before.

Keeping their fear in mind, I assured them that I had been at the bedside of other people who had died and that Mark's dying was normal. I suggested that we sit quietly with Mark so that he could die, if this was the time. Nick, Mark's parents, a friend, and I sat by Mark, held his hands, and talked quietly to him.

We told Mark that we loved him, that we would stay with him, and that there was no reason to be afraid. If he was ready to go on, he could. Just let it happen. We would be all right. Slowly, Mark's breathing became more peaceful and less frequent. He stopped breathing and died, as he had described in his third interview about how he wanted to die.

Afterward, each of us spent time alone with Mark. Then we hugged each other, cried, and talked about his good death. Mark's mother noted that he had put his financial affairs in order and died before running out of health insurance. She said that he did not want his loved ones to be inconvenienced because of him. The next day, Nick described Mark's death as "splendid."

At the request of Mark's parents and Nick, my husband and I went to Mark's memorial service. People and flowers packed the auditorium. Mark's picture stood on a table by his ashes. After beautiful music, Nick went to the lectern and said with tears in his eyes, "I don't want you to think that I am depressed. Mark had a good death. He died like he wanted to die."

Then, as planned by Mark before dying, the leader of the service began to read Mark's third interview, as described above. First, she read the question that I had asked, and then she gave Mark's answer. As Mark's words filled the auditorium, a hush fell over the crowd. People seemed to feel comforted as they listened to Mark's gift to them. Afterward, the leader asked me and other friends of Mark to say a few words. Then she urged each person to take a handful of daffodil bulbs from baskets in back and plant them in memory of Mark.

After Mark's death, Nick called me periodically to say that he felt good even though he missed Mark. Mark's parents sent me a card saying, "We will never forget your love and support the night he left us. Was something very special." The next spring, the daffodils that I had planted in my front yard bloomed.

Commentary

The PWAs said that their fears about dying were at the core of their conflict. They explained why they were afraid to die. First, death would cheat them out of a long life with their loved ones. As Claudia explained, "Dying is scary because I'm too young." Second, the PWAs did not know when and how they would die. "It's the uncertainty that gets you," said Jack. "I don't know how long I will live. My supreme fear has been a loss of mental faculties."

A third reason for fearing death was uncertainty about what happens afterward. Some PWAs feared that death is the end. "Not existing is frightening," said Sally. Other PWAs wondered whether and how to prepare for an afterlife. "If there isn't life after death, why try in this life?" asked Robert. Margaret questioned, "How do I make peace with God so I'm not afraid of dying and I'll go to heaven?"

For several reasons, the significant persons feared the death of their loved ones. They were uncertain about how their loved ones would die and what to do to help them. They did not want their loved ones to be in pain, and they themselves did not want to be left alone. They would need to start a new life. As James put it, "Dealing with his death is so painful that it lowers my self-esteem. I feel more susceptible to hurt. I withhold myself from other people in order to protect myself, and my self-esteem suffers."

The participants said that friends, health care personnel, and society gave them little help to effectively resolve their ethical problems involving death. As illustrated by the story about Mark's death, most people have not seen someone actually die because in

Western society deaths primarily take place in an institution rather than at home. Families may not know how to help a member die at home because they are accustomed to letting health care personnel handle death.

For the most part, health care personnel are poorly prepared to help PWAs and their loved ones, who are often their own age, deal with ethical problems regarding death. They may be able to perform appropriate treatments, but they may not know how to facilitate a good death. As Tony put it, "Nurses and doctors are trained to make people well, but they aren't trained to help people face up to death."

Societal debates about death do not focus on how to facilitate someone to experience a good death. Instead, discussion revolves around technical, impersonal terms—withholding or withdrawing life-sustaining treatment, euthanasia, expiration, futility, prolongation of dying, killing, and assisted suicide (Battin, 1992; Brock, 1992; Danis & Churchill, 1991; Faber-Langendoen & Bartels, 1992; Freeman, 1992; Gold, Jablonski, Christensen, Shapiro, & Schiedermayer, 1990; Wolf, 1992; Wurzbach, 1990).

The participants said that they wanted to resolve their ethical problems in a manner that would facilitate a good death for them or their loved ones. Figure 6.1 illustrates what they said concerning characteristics of a good death. Their stories suggest that research-based programs are needed to educate society, health care personnel, and dying individuals and their loved ones about how to die well.

Additional research would develop knowledge about the dying process and reduce some uncertainty and mystery surrounding death. With increased understanding, people may feel less fearful and talk openly about dying. As Chris put it, "My mother gave me straight answers, and that demystified death."

Research-based education would help shift the focus of societal debates away from abstract analysis using impersonal, technical terms. Instead, public discourse would take into account the personal side of dying and how to facilitate a good death (Loewy, 1992; Meier, 1992). This change in perspective itself may result in effective resolutions to many of society's ethical problems about death, such as if and when euthanasia and suicide are justified, and how far health care personnel should go in facilitating a good death.

ACCEPTANCE: "Something about death that give me a sweetness, when I know it's going to be all right."

VIEW OF DEATH AS PART OF LIFE: "I view death as an open door, not the end of life."

PERSONAL CONTROL: "I don't want to be kept alive by life support."

DIGNITY, NOT SUFFERING: "She asked me to help her go home (to die) with dignity and without long suffering."

PEACE WITH PEOPLE: "You'll feel better if you've been a good person who is nice to other people."

PEACE WITH GOD/HIGHER POWER AND BELIEF IN A PLEASANT AFTERLIFE: "I'm trying to live the life God wants me to live so I have a good death and go to heaven."

LOVED ONES BY ONE'S SIDE: "I would like to be at home with my lover, and my mother and father."

Figure 6.1. Characteristics of a Good Death

No longer would death and bereavement services be relegated to hospice care, but they would become part of mainstream health care (O'Neil, 1989). Health care personnel would become attuned to their own experience of mortality and loss, so that they develop comfort with discussions about dying. They would learn to assess the meaning of living and dying for someone who is dying and facilitate the person's decision making, resulting in a good death (Nokes & Carver, 1991; Phillips, 1992).

The participants' stories suggest what an individual can do to facilitate the experience of a good death for someone. Peter treated his lover with affection and goodness. Meagan maintained a hopeful, optimistic attitude, doing helpful things for her boyfriend. Tony came to accept the increasing disability and inevitable death of his wife, and he carried out her wishes regarding how she wanted to die. Sometimes the most effective strategy is to help the dying person's loved one. Jeffrey's physician could not do much for Jeffrey, but because he nurtured Sonia she was able to nurture her son.

Planning for death facilitates a good death. "We have been talking with his parents about how he wants to die," James said. "We will discuss his death with his doctor and take care of the legal problems." Use of health care proxies and advance directives can maximize an individual's control of decision making about treatment options (Schwarz, 1992).

When the actual death draws near, being there facilitates a good death. "Dying is meant to be a shared experience," wrote Carlos. "You step closer to the truth." Being present provides the opportunity to let go and help the dying person to let go, too. Sonia said that she gave Jeffrey permission to die, and he gave his mother permission to go on with her life.

James put it well when he described how he was helping his lover to die well, which he eventually did. "I want to help him die with peace, not anger," he explained. "To have a sense that he's done everything he needs to. That he accepts dying. I want to help him have a sense of God or higher power. I want to say to him, 'You can go. I can carry on. I want you to be happy.' I want him to know he's loved and comforted into his death."

In summary, the participants' stories suggest the need for society, health care personnel, and individuals to shift from technical, impersonal analyses of death to personal discussions about what a good death is and how to facilitate it. This change in focus itself may lead to effective resolutions to societal and individual ethical problems involving death.

7

Ethical Problems Involving Discrimination

Stigmatizing PWAs creates complicated ethical problems for AIDS-impacted individuals, health care personnel, and society. Historically, society has discriminated against men who have sex with men, persons who inject drugs, and people of color, whose behavior may put them at risk for HIV disease (Grossman, 1991). The World Health Organization (WHO) described three epidemics: the silent pandemic of HIV disease, the clinical disease of AIDS, and the widespread fearful reaction to AIDS (National Center for Nursing Research, 1990). Because of hysteria about AIDS, PWAs have been denied housing, schooling, insurance, health care, employment, and even burial (Trenk, 1989).

On December 2, 1988, Surgeon General C. Everett Koop startled a national audience of health care personnel by proposing that AIDS be viewed like any other chronic illness (Blendon & Donelan, 1990). This statement raised the question about whether PWAs' ethical problems are similar to ethical problems experienced by persons with other chronic illnesses such as heart disease and cancer, and if not, why? Although research has not been reported in answer to this question, the participants' stories suggest a fundamental difference regarding the ethical problems of PWAs.

The participants described ethical problems that may be like ethical problems related to other chronic illnesses. For example, persons with heart disease and cancer may experience the kinds of ethical problems addressed in the chapter on chronic illness. In addition, they may face ethical problems involving alcohol and drugs, death, discrimination, finances and business, health care, personhood, relationships, service, and sexuality. However, persons with other chronic illnesses probably are not confronted by the painful and extensive discrimination that the participants described and that is well-documented in the literature (Blendon & Donelan, 1990; Crimp, 1988; Watney, 1987).

Thirteen PWAs (4 women and 9 men) and two significant persons (1 woman and 1 man) specifically described ethical problems involving discrimination: "Should I avoid people even though I need them?" "Should I be honest or secretive about AIDS?" "Should I be honest or secretive about being gay and having AIDS?" "Is it right to lie to avoid discrimination?" "Is it right to be prejudiced toward homosexuals even though I believe in equality?" "Should I tell travel authorities that I have AIDS even though they may discriminate against me?"

"Should I Avoid People Even Though I Need Them?"

JANET

Janet, a PWA who identified herself as "White and of French and German ancestry," questioned if she should avoid people even though she needed them. "I think about AIDS all the time and what will happen to me," Janet said. "You don't want to talk about AIDS because you don't know how people may react. They talk to you, but it ain't that close contact like before. They are prejudiced. They say they ain't, but they don't take time to talk to you. God, you're a human being, too. You feel alone. Who is there that really cares?"

Although Janet had not resolved her conflict, she said, "I talk to the AIDS educator. I haven't talked to other people." She rationalized, "The AIDS educator cares. Other people don't understand."

ANDREW

Andrew, an "African-American" PWA, described conflict about whether he should avoid people even though he needed them. "My family would stick by me," he said, "but I'm afraid I'll lose my friends because of AIDS. If I get sick, they would drift off and become distant. It would hurt something terrible. That's the biggest thing I fear, because I wouldn't want nobody to treat me different than the way they do now."

"If they treat me differently," Andrew resolved, "I'll tell them, 'Don't treat me like this. You're not going to catch it from hanging out with me.' "

He reasoned, "I value friendships. Without nobody to talk to, you could go crazy. I wouldn't want to be alone, not with AIDS, because you shouldn't be so. It's easier to face life with friends. Then you have somebody to help you understand what's going on with you. A lonely life isn't as good a life as life with friends. If you're lonely, it will make the disease worse."

ISAAC

Isaac, a PWA, identified himself as a "gay African American." To protect his confidentiality, we met secretly at an agency. Like Janet and Andrew, he described conflict about whether he should avoid people even though he needed them.

"How should I deal with prejudice involving AIDS?" Isaac asked. "It's hard to be yourself when you are treated negatively. In such a racist and mixed-up society, people assume that someone of color is infected. I have a right to confidentiality. Who can I talk to? Who can I trust? If someone needs to know that I have AIDS, what are the repercussions?"

Isaac described his resolution to his conflict. "I try to live as normally as possible," he said, "being careful about who I talk to. I have learned a lot about confidentiality, what it means and how the information is used against you or for you."

"The prejudice comes from fear or lack of understanding," Isaac rationalized. "Society closes the door on people who are infected.

It's important to think about how to share information in a correct way. You need to know how to survive and live comfortably with AIDS and have the assurance that you're OK and information you end up giving is not used against you."

ANNE

I met Anne, an "African-American" PWA, at an agency so that her children would not hear the interview. For the second interview, I went to her home. Anne, too, questioned whether to avoid people even though she needed them.

"You tell somebody that you have AIDS, and they reject you," Anne said. "The person you thought would accept, don't. You want to say, 'Please don't turn your back on me. I need you.' One of the greatest fears beside having AIDS is to be rejected and not loved. My second mom don't want me in her house, and it hurted me deep 'cuz I love her. She's afraid that she will get the virus. It's painful, and I cry."

Describing her resolution to her conflict, Anne said, "You hesitant to talk about AIDS. With my second mom, if I sit down to think on the hurt, I will end up in the hospital and won't be able to take care of my family. I say that it hurt, so I faced it and try not to let it hurt so much. With rejection, you got to pull yourself up and keep a positive mind. You got to love yourself enough to know that you going to make it."

"Rejection is like taking a suicide pill," Anne said explaining her rationale, "not totally dead but cut you off or limit you. It's something you have to deal with besides everything else. A lot of time, that's what people have, rejection. It cause you to go down, to weaken. It suppress the immune system, the mind, the body. People reject because they don't understand what rejection do to you."

"Love soothe you," Anne said. "Love is warmth and understanding, having somebody hug me or pat my hand, tell me that HIV is like cancer or other diseases. Somebody to bear you up, to motivate you. Love do not see a fault. Love do not make you back up but bring you forth. It's going the extra mile. We should show more love. I cry tons because it hurts me when I see people being rejected. With love, medicine that the doctor give you can bring more healing."

"Should I Be Honest or Secretive About AIDS?"

STAN

Stan, who had hemophilia and was "of mostly German ancestry," asked to meet me in my office so that no one else would know about his AIDS diagnosis. He questioned whether he should be honest or secretive about having AIDS.

"I want to be open," Stan began, "but because of the stigma surrounding AIDS I lead a double life. If you say you've got AIDS, people assume that you got it through IV drugs or you're gay. I'm neither. I'd like to shout, 'Look, you moron, it's not my fault. I'm fine in terms of morals.' But I can't do that because it's counterproductive. I don't like keeping deep, dark secrets. AIDS is one of those things it shouldn't make any difference."

"Does the medical community have a right to know that I have AIDS, or should I just remind them of precautions for HIV infection?" Stan asked. "Should my wife and I tell our children? If it gets around, the school may discriminate against them. Do my wife's parents have a right to know? It would hurt their restaurant business. How should I deal with my friends? I don't want them to know in case it would hurt me and my children. Should I tell the people at work or a potential employer? AIDS has not compromised my ability to do the job. It may keep me from getting promotions and salary increases. Do I have responsibilities that go beyond my own life and position because people depend on me?"

Stan described his resolution to his conflict. "When first diagnosed," he said, "I thought I had only 6 months to live and I should tell people so they could take over my responsibilities. My wife cautioned me about more people knowing than necessary. I cut the list of people that I intended to talk to. I can survive this for awhile, so there's no need to tell everyone yet."

"We resolve who to tell on a case-by-case basis," Stan continued. "I remind medical personnel about precautions for HIV infection so they won't become infected themselves. I told my dentist. My doctors and nurse know. So that my kids won't find out, I get my AIDS medications at a different pharmacy than other medications. We haven't told my wife's family, but I don't chop salad vegetables anymore in their restaurant. We have told only a few friends and people at work."

"I'd like to throttle people who tell AIDS jokes," Stan said, "but, usually, I don't say anything and go on. The other screaming times are people who are stupid about modes of HIV transmission, when I can't change what they think."

"First," Stan rationalized, "don't hurt anybody, such as myself or family, physically or emotionally. If you can do anything on top of that, do so. I tell people according to the seriousness of their need to know. I don't lie, but I don't tell the whole truth. I don't feel any requirement to explain to strangers. It's your responsibility to tell medical people that you're HIV-infected. They need to know in order to safeguard their health. They don't need to know anything other than to take precautions for HIV."

PHILLIP

Like Stan, Phillip, who described himself as "White," also had hemophilia and AIDS. He, too, described conflict about whether to be honest or secretive about AIDS.

"When I found out that I was HIV-positive," Phillip said, "my wife and I decided not to tell anyone and not to have children. Why worry or hurt anyone? If people feel sorry for me, it weakens me. After I was diagnosed with AIDS, we had a real struggle. We wanted to tell people that would be beneficial. We weren't strong enough to handle this by ourselves. We needed people telling me that I'll make it."

Explaining his resolution to his conflict, Phillip said, "We called my mother, my wife's parents, my brothers and sisters, some friends," he said. "It started mushrooming until everybody found out. I had a big problem with all of them knowing. I didn't want to be a person that people would not shake hands with or talk to or eat with. Why do they have to tell everyone? It took several months for me to accept that they know. But that hasn't been enough support. We are wondering who else to tell and how."

"I tell professionals, doctors and nurses who work on me and need to protect themselves, that I have AIDS," Phillip said. "It's hard to discuss. I had a toothache and delayed going to a dentist because I didn't want the hassle about AIDS. Finally, my wife called the dentist and said I had AIDS. She asked if he would treat me. The dentist said, 'No,' and referred me to another dentist who said he would not treat me. We contacted the University School of Dentistry and had my tooth worked on there. They made me feel welcome. The head of the Dentistry School called the two dentists to say that was wrong and there should be universal precautions throughout the dental industry. For awhile, I felt like a social outcast, a leper. Now, I could tell a dentist, 'I've got AIDS and do you want to work on me or not? If you don't feel comfortable, I'll go to someone else.' "

"I decided not to go to my high school reunion because I looked sick," he said. "My family still live in that town. A lady I worked for there stood up in church and said to pray for me because I have AIDS. The president of our class stood up at the banquet and said to pray for me because I'm ill. Everybody knew that I had AIDS by the end of the weekend. I received a letter from my class and a check to go away for a weekend at a hotel. I was touched by that. I drove through town, but I'll never go back. Why go to that conflict situation if I don't have to? They would feel sorry for me and treat me different."

Phillip explained his rationale for his resolution. "From reading the Bible," he said, "I realized I was being selfish not to tell people that work on me that I have AIDS. I don't want anybody else to be affected by my terminal illness because I was too proud or too stubborn to tell them. Human life is more important than my feelings. I trust in God that He will provide for me, and He has. By opening up to people, I got support that gave me the strength to fight to live."

ALBERTA

Alberta, a PWA, said that she was "half Black and half White." Like Stan and Phillip, she described conflict about whether to be honest or secretive about having AIDS.

"I wouldn't want to tell nobody what I had," Alberta said. "That's scary. It's embarrassing to tell somebody, 'I got AIDS,' because that's a deadly disease. People be thinking, 'What the hell was she doing? Are they passing that disease that she picked up?' I'm sure my boyfriend don't want to tell people what we got. You don't know who to talk to about it."

"I told my sister and my oldest daughter and my best friend," she said about her resolution. "That's the only people. My boyfriend knows because I got the test first, and then he had to get it. As soon as that guy told me I had AIDS, I couldn't wait to find me a support group. I went to the support group, and it's great."

"Soon as you get something like this," Alberta explained her rationale for her resolution, "go to a support group because you'll go crazy if you don't tell nobody about it. You got to get yourself help. It's easier to talk to people you don't know because you can come out and say anything. You can get it off your chest and feel comfortable."

LEAH

Leah, a significant person and "Caucasian," described conflict about whether to be honest or secretive about AIDS. "Should I tell my parents that my boyfriend has AIDS?" she asked. "It's unfair not to tell them. What if they find out, and I didn't tell them first? They would be upset and perhaps think that I didn't love them enough to tell them. If something happened, they would have to deal with everything at once. If I tell them, they can give support."

"But I don't have the guts to tell my parents," said Leah. "They might say that I can't go out with my boyfriend any more because they don't want me to be hurt. If I tell them, they will go through the same thing that I'm going through, crying all the time, feeling depressed and helpless. They know him, like him, and think that he is a healthy young man. If they only knew."

"How should I tell my parents?" asked Leah. "I want to tell them in such as way as to get them to support me in my decision to stay with my boyfriend. I worry about whether I should do it one way or another. Should we go to their home? Should we tell them when we get there or when we are leaving? How to tell them is a no-win situation."

"What other people besides my parents should we tell?" Leah asked. "I'm good at hiding things. I'm afraid of people knowing too much about me. Is it selfish to tell people so they can give support? The news will give them pain. I don't want to tell people who will try to change my mind about staying with him."

Leah described her resolution. "I haven't told my parents, even though I should," she said. "Before we get formally engaged, we will tell them for sure. I drop little hints to let them know. I feel bad about hiding this because it takes a toll on me. I tell myself that they don't have to know. It's not life-threatening to them or anything. Then I feel better."

"For a year, we didn't tell my identical twin sister with whom I live," Leah said. "But she found out anyway, and we felt stupid for not telling her. We told my manager, because I have to miss work sometimes to go to the hospital to be with my boyfriend. We told our closest friends who give us support. We haven't told friends who aren't close to us."

Leah rationalized, "Telling someone about my boyfriend having AIDS is giving part of myself away, and I want to give it to somebody I can trust. Trust means that I feel confident that the person is not going to tell another person, use the information against me, or reject me. People I trust give me love even if they disagree with me. We don't try to hurt each other. Only good friends need to know that he has AIDS. Why hurt other people with the news? They can't do anything. We tell people who will give us support, and we need this support."

"Should I Be Honest or Secretive About Being Gay and Having AIDS?"

RYAN

Ryan, identifying himself as "Anglo-Saxon," described conflict about whether he should be honest or secretive about being gay and having AIDS. "What is the right way to come out as a PWA?" he asked. "I want to live my life in an open, honest way, but my parents have said to hide who I am from my extended family. I feel responsible to obey my parents so that my extended family won't say I am gay because they were inadequate parents and brought me up wrong."

"Because I hide who I am from my extended family," Ryan said, "I feel alienated from them, and I cannot draw on their support. I am more comfortable being around my friends who know the full scope of my life. My relationships with my relatives are superficial and unsatisfying. I feel bad about myself because I am withholding information. Even though my relatives may feel pain and be critical, I want them to know so that I can be honest with them."

"I have been honest with my parents, staff, and friends about being gay and having AIDS," Ryan said about his resolution to his conflict. "Now I can talk to them. I was touched by the compassionate reaction of my staff and friends."

"I have not told my extended family," Ryan continued, "but I avoid being dishonest with them. I may select nonjudgmental relatives to tell, without telling my parents first. I would write them extensive letters about who I am and ask them to be an advocate for me with the rest of the family. If my parents hear that I told some members of my extended family, I will deal with that situation then."

Explaining his rationale for his resolution, Ryan said, "I wanted my staff and friends to hear it from me because I was going to need their support desperately. I want to be honest with my extended family. Being gay and having AIDS is something I cannot change. I want to be part of the family, not alienated anymore. I think they will feel compassion for me. When the time comes, they can give support to my parents. Acknowledging the truth could be enriching for my parents and extended family. Even though they may experience pain at first, they may become more compassionate people."

JOSH

Josh, "Caucasian" and a significant person for Ryan, described conflict about whether to be honest or secretive about Ryan being gay and having AIDS. "I can't deal with AIDS by myself," said Josh, "so I need to tell other people in order to obtain their support. I can't count on my family for support. Because I'm giving him all my love, I don't have the energy to deal with the complexities of other relationships and with people who aren't fully supportive. How should I be the person I want to be and obtain needed support from other people without depleting my own energy?"

Josh resolved, "I will selectively tell other people that my lover has AIDS in order to obtain support. I will avoid telling people who will criticize me. I will tell people in such a way as to find out which people I can depend on and when." He reasoned, "I need the support of other people. I need to know on whom I can depend."

"Is It Right to Lie to Avoid Discrimination?"

LARRY

Larry, a PWA and "White," described conflict about whether to lie about his AIDS medication in order to hide his diagnosis. "I don't want people at work to know that I have AIDS because they will treat me differently," he said. "I don't want their sympathy. I know lying is wrong, but is it all right to lie so they won't find out that I have AIDS?"

"I've only told a few people at work that I have AIDS, and I don't want anyone else to know," said Larry, describing his resolution. "One day I was mixing my medication. A guy asked what it is. He doesn't know I am ill. I don't care for him to know, either. I said it's an antacid. I actually lied."

Larry rationalized, "It's more important to be treated normal than to tell a little lie. I know instinctively that lying is wrong. You've got to tell the truth whenever possible. Most people know when they aren't telling the truth. In this case, I felt that lying was all right, and God forgave me. I don't feel good about lying, but it's more important not to hurt myself than to tell a white lie. There's that balance thing."

"Is It Right to Be Prejudiced Toward Homosexuals Even Though I Believe in Equality?"

EUGENE

Eugene identified himself as "White and heterosexual," explaining that he became HIV-infected from a blood product used to treat his hemophilia. He described conflict about whether it was right to be prejudiced toward homosexuals.

"I can't accept homosexuals," Eugene said. "I don't believe that God wants homosexuals to have sex in that way. It's a learned trait that's not right. Being in contact with them isn't good for me because it gives me too much conflict. I've got enough to deal with without that, too."

"The gay men at the clinic asked me to be in their support group," Eugene continued. "I said, 'No.' I'm too angry at them because I have AIDS. Gay sex was one of the major transmissions. If people weren't gay, maybe I wouldn't have AIDS. I know it's wrong to blame homosexuals. I could have gotten it from anybody that contributed blood. I should accept homosexuals as people like I am, even though they're messed up. I'm uneasy about being angry at them because they're children of God, whether they believe in God or not."

"I want to help a gay person if I can," resolved Eugene, "but I try not to be socially exposed to that type of person. I may get counseling to straighten out my feelings about them so that I don't blame them anymore. I want to be able to accept them as humans. It's hard. I've gotta stop being so closed-minded."

"It's wrong to be angry at another child of God because we're all one," Eugene rationalized. "We all have a chance for eternal life. They are as good as me or anybody else. I don't have a right to judge anybody else for what they do. They've got to deal with that themselves. When it comes to Judgment Day, you have to explain, and the way that you act on earth determines what happens then."

JOEL

Joel, who identified himself as "White and heterosexual," said that he had become HIV-infected from a blood product used to treat his hemophilia. He, like Eugene, described conflict about whether it was right to be prejudiced toward homosexuals.

"People who know that I have AIDS see me as heterosexual," Joel said. "No one thinks I'm bisexual. In college, some people may have thought that I'm gay. I don't consider homosexuality to be natural. It's fine as long as it doesn't affect my life. How should I deal with society's prejudice toward gay people because I have AIDS which is associated with gays? I'm bothered by bigotry."

Describing his resolution, he said, "I'm a firm believer in equality and run my personal and professional life accordingly. This value comes from my family, which is good, old WASP."

Joel explained his rationale for his resolution. "Each person has individual rights whether male/female, White/Black or whatever," he said. "You should not abridge those rights and privileges for something trivial. It is logical not to discriminate against somebody based on what they were born with or their beliefs as long as it doesn't affect what you're doing. People have the right of sameness, the right to do whatever every other group can do. There's no reason this person should be prohibited from doing something that any other person is allowed to do by laws or the moral structure. A person should not be prevented from going into certain professions, except from a lack of innate ability."

"Should I Tell Travel Authorities That I Have AIDS Even Though They May Discriminate Against Me?"

PAUL

Paul, who identified himself as "White," said that he had both hemophilia and AIDS. Concerned about confidentiality, he asked to participate in the research anonymously. He described conflict about whether he should tell travel authorities that he had AIDS even though they might discriminate against him.

"Should I disclose to travel authorities that I have AIDS?" Paul asked. "Should I avoid infecting the populace in countries where I travel? How should I safely discard syringes that I need for medications without notifying the travel authorities that I have AIDS? When I travel, should I break my monogamy and engage in sin? Should I avoid travel to protect my own health?"

"When I travel," Paul said, describing his resolution to his conflict, "I don't disclose that I have AIDS. When I recently went to a conference, I went ahead and no questions were asked. I don't lie, but I don't tell the whole truth."

"I dispose of syringes for my medications without infecting anyone and without disclosing that I have AIDS," Paul continued. "I ask where medical treatment is. I look into what documentation I need to cart syringes with me. I don't interact with the populace in a way to transmit the virus. I am firm in my monogamy and don't participate in sin."

Explaining his rationale, Paul said, "Since I'm not going to interact with the populace in a way to transmit the virus, the authorities don't need to know that I have AIDS. My wife and I were raised to be firm in our monogamy. I'm not going to contaminate anyone. I don't want to hurt myself or other people, even if it takes extra effort. I am more worried about traveling to another country because of my own health than because they might find out that I have AIDS. Some countries have abysmal water and sanitation systems. It's my problem if I fall sick in the country, and I have to deal with the consequences."

"My sense of responsibility to society comes from my religion and the way I was raised," Paul said. "I have a deep faith in God.

The moral structures in the different religions are all the same, even in ones with no identifiable being. The fine points of the religions are a little different. I don't buy a strict, it-is-written in the Bible, type of thing. There's nothing in there about syringes and telling somebody about AIDS. You have to answer these questions in the context of how you were raised and the religion."

MARILYN

Marilyn, a PWA, identified herself as "Hispanic, Black, Russian, and American Indian." Like Paul, she described conflict about whether she should tell travel authorities that she had AIDS even though they might discriminate against her.

"I want to go to Europe," Marilyn said. "I can't go out of the country because they have some law that if you have AIDS, you can't. I could travel and not tell them because I can't see them giving everybody a blood test that comes into the country. But I'm afraid that if I went, they'd find out in some way, capture me, and put me in jail."

Marilyn had not resolved her conflict. "I don't know what to do about travel," she said. "Right now I'm not traveling." She reasoned, "I don't want to go to jail for the rest of my life. If I don't travel, I don't have to risk going to jail in another country."

Commentary

The participants' stories illustrate the pain of stigmatization. As Anne put it, "You tell somebody that you have AIDS, and they reject you. Rejection is like taking a suicide pill, not totally dead but cut you off or limit you. It's something you have to deal with besides everything else. It suppress the immune system, the mind, the body."

No matter what their situation, the participants said that they had experienced discrimination. "If you say you've got AIDS," said Stan, "people assume that you got it through IV drugs or you're gay. I'm neither." They questioned whether lying about AIDS was justified to avoid discrimination.

Craving emotional support, the participants wanted to tell other people about having AIDS or loving someone with AIDS. They feared rejection, however, and hesitated divulging this information. Consequently, they felt isolated from other people. As Janet said, "You don't want to talk about AIDS because you don't know how people may react. You feel alone. Who is there that really cares?"

In various ways, the participants resolved their ethical problems involving discrimination. They reached out for help by joining a support group, turning to God, and carefully selecting confidantes who would support them. Rather than become bitter, they tried to develop positive thinking. They took steps to live in as "normal" a manner as possible.

Wary about confiding in health care personnel, some PWAs divulged their diagnosis, whereas other PWAs simply reminded them to use universal precautions. Many of the participants led duplicitous lives. As Stan put it, "I want to be open, but because of the stigma surrounding AIDS I lead a double life."

At the core of the participants' ethical problems is conflict between the public good and individual rights. AIDS has heightened this conflict because of society's negative attitudes about homosexuality and about intravenous drug use by poor persons of color who live in the inner city. Many people blame PWAs for becoming infected, and they do not want public funds to be used to help them. They fear becoming HIV-infected themselves, and they react with hostility to PWAs. Even some participants struggled with negative attitudes about homosexuality and intravenous drug use.

Conflict between the public good and individual rights can be seen in questions about the right way to curb HIV transmission. Some authors favor mandatory testing and reporting, closing of gay bathhouses, and even quarantine, claiming that such activities would not discriminate but would merely implement traditional public health practices that have been used successfully against other contagious diseases. Other authors contend that such activities violate individual rights by leading to discrimination against HIV-infected persons who may be denied housing, employment, insurance, and privacy (Tauer, 1989).

In questions regarding testing for HIV disease, conflict between the public good and individual rights arises. Some authors argue that such testing should be handled like any other test that is ordered at the physician's discretion. Other authors claim that testing for HIV disease should be treated differently because no other illness in recent times has elicited the prejudice that AIDS has (Childress, 1991; Grady, 1992).

Conflict between the public good and individual rights is apparent in questions about programs through which public health officials contact needle-sharing and sex partners of persons who are HIV-infected. The purpose is to notify these persons about their risk for HIV disease, suggest testing, and offer treatment if they are infected. Conflict arises because officials can do little to force HIV-infected persons to reveal their partners, and these programs must depend on trust among officials, persons with HIV disease, and their partners. However, HIV-infected persons and their partners may doubt the confidentiality of the disclosure or the motives of the officials (Gostin, 1987).

The participants' stories suggest strategies for resolving ethical problems involving discrimination. Laws should be enacted that specifically prohibit discrimination toward HIV-infected persons. HIV testing, partner notification, and other public health measures should be used only when their purposes are clear, their results are productive, and individual rights and privacy are protected (Cooper & Weiss, 1989; DePhilippis, Metzger, Woody, & Navaline, 1992; Murphy, 1991c; Stein, 1991; Stoddard & Rieman, 1990). Even if health care personnel do not approve of the behavior of some persons at risk for or having HIV disease, they should provide quality care for them. The government should support research to develop and evaluate programs for respectfully helping people to change their high-risk behavior (Cleary et al., 1991). Research-based, confidential counseling should be provided before and after testing for HIV disease at sites where clients are seen for other reasons. Using language that their clients understand, counselors would talk about the risk of infection, ways in which the risk can be reduced or eliminated, notification of partners, and treatment options (Hinman, 1991). To avoid AIDS hysteria, scientists, health care personnel, public officials, activists, and journalists should publish timely, informative, responsible publications about AIDS (Colby & Cook, 1991; Nelkin, 1991).

Certainly, the primary way to resolve ethical problems involving discrimination toward AIDS-impacted individuals is to change from the current military metaphor to a caring metaphor. Too often, the goal of curbing HIV transmission is viewed as winning a war, dividing society into two camps: persons who are at risk for or have HIV disease and those who are not. The former persons are the enemy, and they must be controlled or conquered. Caring focuses on building trust and developing communal efforts out of concern for AIDS-impacted individuals (Bennett, 1990; Childress, 1991). Through caring, conflict between the public good and individual rights can be more effectively resolved.

A caring metaphor would be more likely than a military metaphor to encourage persons who are at high risk for or have HIV disease to stop engaging in duplicity and take steps to prevent HIV transmission. Caring would facilitate their work with public health officials and health care personnel to develop legal initiatives and treatment options (DePhilippis et al., 1992). In a caring atmosphere, these persons would be better able to build satisfying relationships that contribute to healthy behavior.

In summary, the participants said that they yearned for caring relationships, but because of stigmatization they often felt alone. Explaining the importance of caring, Anne said, "Love is warmth and understanding, having somebody hug me or pat my hand, tell me that HIV is like cancer or other diseases. Somebody to bear you up, to motivate you. With love, medicine that the doctor give you can bring more healing." A caring society develops creative solutions to promote the public good while safeguarding individual rights.

8

Ethical Problems Involving
Finances and Business

Being chronically ill with HIV disease is expensive, not just in terms of health care but also day-to-day living. Most PWAs live in poverty. If they are not poor before being diagnosed with HIV disease, they frequently become poor as their disability removes them from the labor market and the costs of their care exhaust their assets. Society's history of discriminating against PWAs compounds their socioeconomic plight (Vladeck, 1989). As their financial and business situation deteriorates, PWAs experience difficult ethical problems.

Like PWAs, society must deal with ethical problems involving finances and business in regard to HIV disease. As more persons develop AIDS, attention is turning to financial ramifications. Society must determine which services to provide for persons who are infected and affected by HIV disease and how to pay for them. Economists can predict the average cost of services for PWAs. However, these direct expenses pale in comparison with the loss to society of the potential economic productivity of relatively young people whose lives end prematurely. Add indirect costs generated by disruptions in social and economic activity caused by the fear of contagion, and the resulting price tag is astronomical (Fox & Thomas, 1990; Vladeck, 1989).

The PWAs in this research told me that their occupations were: actor, AIDS activist, banker, car washer, choreographer, clergy, community liaison, computer technician, contractor, educator, homemaker, hospital administrator, librarian, machinist, manager, nurse, nurses' aide, paralegal, researcher, salesperson, social worker, student, and waitress. The significant persons' occupations were: architect, technician, student, mother, and food caterer. Because of discrimination or deteriorating health, most of the PWAs said that they no longer worked full time, and they were experiencing the kinds of financial and business difficulties that are documented in the literature about other PWAs (Kass, Faden, Fox, & Dudley, 1991).

Eight PWAs (four women and four men) specifically described ethical problems involving finances and business: "Is it right to engage in illegal activities to make ends meet?" "Should I hold a job for financial and emotional reasons even though it jeopardizes my health?" "Is it right to benefit from AIDS?" "Although I value the expertise of lawyers, should I follow their advice when I don't trust them?" "Should I plan a funeral I can't afford or be satisfied with a county-paid funeral?"

"Is It Right to Engage in Illegal Activities to Make Ends Meet?"

CATHERINE

Catherine, a PWA and "dance choreographer," attended school in between jobs. A high school dropout, she described conflict about whether to engage in illegal activities to make ends meet.

"I'm not sick enough to get money from the government," Catherine said, "but I'm not well enough to work. I have to rely on welfare. After paying my rent, I don't have enough left for the month. I'm a vegetarian, and what they give me for food only lasts for 2 weeks. The other 2 weeks I don't have no money unless I go do something to get money. How should I make ends meet? I could go strip out of town. I could clean up if I was a prostitute. I'd have a car, a house, and everything."

Catherine described her resolution to her conflict. "I go strip out of town," she said. "I get to that point where I need to have money. I don't let myself go to the extreme that I might if I was younger, like prostitution. I don't like to do prostitution." She paused and then said, "Maybe, one day, I might get forced into the situation."

"They're putting you in this miserable state," Catherine rationalized, "and you have no reason to live. It's a way of making sure somebody dies faster. I'm young. I can't live without money and be happy. I need money to do all the things I want to do before I die. I'd like to fly in an airplane, travel, have a car, be able to get to the hospital and to school, see my family, go to the library and drum classes, to take dance classes to keep my body healthy."

PEGGY

Peggy, a PWA and former "waitress," said that she lived "on welfare," which was not sufficient for her needs. Like Catherine, she described conflict about whether it was right to engage in illegal activities to make ends meet.

"It's not bad being on welfare," Peggy said, "but they don't give you nothing. I want to improve my health, but I don't have the money to buy good food to do that. You don't make it if you work or don't work. If you got a job, you've got to let them know. If you don't let them know, you get in trouble. If you do let them know, they take it out of your check. They're like the police. You don't have no privacy."

"I want to go steal," Peggy said. "You don't get much money from shoplifting or writing bad checks. So I'd rob me a bank. That's taking a big project. But it's having a lot of money, too. Getting away with it is another thing. My luck, I'd get caught before I even get out of the bank because I'd freak out. I see the cops, I get scared. I'm scared of guns, so I probably wouldn't make a good bank robber. If I got shot by the police, I wouldn't be able to spend the money."

Peggy resolved, "I live on government assistance and don't do any stealing—right now. I wouldn't let nobody know if I was. I'd hurry up and do it and get it over with."

"It's not going to happen that I will get more money," reasoned Peggy. "So I try to live on a little amount of money. The only reason why I don't steal is I don't want to die in jail. I'm scared of jail. I've been in jail before for writing bad checks. I know how bad jail can be. That's the only thing that stops me from doing anything wrong. But if I get desperate for money or ill so I'm going to die pretty soon, the fear of jail ain't going to stop me.

"I want to get some money for my kids," continued Peggy. "If I ever robbed a bank, I would give each of my kids half the money so they would be able to start a life when they get older. So they won't have to scrape and scramble and be on welfare."

"Should I Hold a Job for Financial and Emotional Reasons Even Though It Jeopardizes My Health?"

STEVE

Steve said that before being diagnosed with AIDS he had worked full time as a nurse. Like Catherine and Peggy, his income now was limited. He described conflict about whether he should hold a job for financial and emotional reasons even though working full time could jeopardize his health.

"There is no mechanism for me to do graduated or part-time disability," Steve said. "Either I have to work full time, which physically I can't do, or be totally disabled in order to pay my bills. To be disabled, you have to give up your assets, and you end up in poverty. If I do that, how should I make enough money to meet my needs but not lose my disability benefits?"

"Should I give up private insurance and just take county and state assistance?" Steve asked. "And how do I do that? Should I become ungarnishable, and how? How can I keep from reporting my income? How should I deal with my lack of information about disability options? They give me one number to call, and then they can only talk about one thing. They send me someplace else."

"Now that I have learned information that would make things easier for other people," Steve asked, "should I educate them or concentrate on myself? How effective can I be if I'm not taking care of myself? It's a constant ethical problem."

Describing his resolution to his conflict, Steve said, "I chose total disability over jeopardizing my health. I have Medicare, and I'm on the state plan for people who aren't insured because of a preexisting condition. I went bankrupt, got rid of any assets, and only work so much in order to maintain my disability benefits. I don't report most of my income. I learned as much about disability benefits as I could. I educate people about disability benefits on a case-by-case basis as long as I don't jeopardize my own health."

He reasoned, "The disability system is an ethical nightmare, which I hate. There should be informational seminars or something to teach people how to use the services they're getting. I don't see how it can be cost-effective if you don't allow people to actualize their potential and give them resources to get back on their feet. It seems stupid for me to waste my time. People facing that situation would rather give up and get what they get as opposed to learning what they can take advantage of."

LISA

Lisa, a PWA and computer programmer, described conflict about whether to continue in her job for financial and emotional reasons even though working full time jeopardized her health.

"Before quitting my job," she said, "I didn't know if I should. I'd be sick and then I'd be better. They needed to count on me. They have the right to that. They knew about the AIDS and were supportive."

"There were good reasons to stay in my job," Lisa continued. "I liked having the money. It provided me with insurance. Staying at work provided me with something to do and a good way of self-esteem. There were good reasons to quit my job. It was healthier for me not to be working because it was putting a great deal of strain on me."

"Now that I've quit my job," she said, "there are good reasons to go back to work. My health insurance ends in 2 years. I'm bored, even with the cats here. There are good reasons to stay home. I don't know if it's feasible to get my job back because they're having layoffs. If I go back and get laid off or fired, I may lose everything, which would leave me unemployed, and my only recourse is Social Security, and that's for the shits. I don't need to work since I won't run out of money. I would be the wealthiest if I worked part time."

Lisa described her resolution. "I quit my job a year ago," she said, "and went on long-term disability. I'm making more money than I did when I was working, between long term, Social Security, and a monthly income from something else. I'm leaning away from going back to work." Explaining her rationale, Lisa said, "I've been much healthier since I've stopped working and getting that out of my life. Everything's been fine."

SCOTT

Scott said that he was a banker, even though he had not worked for 2 years because of AIDS. Like Steve and Lisa, he described conflict about whether to hold a job for financial and emotional reasons even though it jeopardized his health.

"When I was diagnosed with AIDS," Scott said, "it wasn't as much of a blow as having a nervous breakdown and losing my job. My employer of 9 years wouldn't let me go back to work even though my psychiatrist felt that I was ready. I'd like to find a full-time job, as long as it doesn't interfere with my illness. If I work part time, I might lose assistance."

"I don't know what to say to people about my work situation," Scott continued. "I can't give them a one-word answer. If I'm not working, there must be a reason. Without a job, I feel like a nonperson, and I'm lonely. You become protective of yourself and defensive. You get invited to a party, and everybody's talking about what they're doing in their jobs and what vacation they're going to take, and I can't relate to those things anymore."

"My disability is about to run out, and I'm worried about ending up on the streets," Scott said. "How could this happen to a guy who had a good job and education? Living on the streets is dangerous. Somebody might attack me. Try to steal what I have. Hurt me physically. Now I view people begging for money in a different way. You don't know what they have been through. They don't have anybody to love them."

"I'm worried about the toll this is taking on my family," Scott went on. "They've been wonderful. But they're constantly worried about me. Then I worry more because I don't want to worry them. I'm worried about living in this group home. It is scary to see people who have the same illness as me die."

"I looked for another job," Scott said about his resolution, "but I couldn't find one that was satisfactory. I find it easier if I don't think too much about it because that will make me depressed. I haven't spent time sharing my feelings because I have to get through a day at a time and take things as they come. I get government assistance, which is basic living. When my disability runs out, I don't know if I would go on the street, or go live with my family, or what."

Scott reasoned, "AIDS has made me more vulnerable than I've been in my life. I was taught by my parents that you pull your weight. Contributing is all I know. I'm not supposed to depend on somebody. I'm supposed to help other people. I want more out of life than I'm getting. I want to be able to take care of myself and have a relationship with somebody. I feel lonely because I don't have many friends now that I'm not working. Life isn't as happy if it's lonely. If you don't have somebody to share accomplishments or be there to talk to, it makes it awful hard. That's another form of rejection and hurts real bad in my heart. If there aren't other people around, I'm not as valuable a person. Other people validate who we are. If they're not there, I don't really exist or I'm not fully who I am."

"If there was any kind of fairness or loyalty," said Scott, "people would be able to get training to work, not necessarily in their field. I'm not bitter. I don't feel I did anything to deserve what's happening. It's not that somebody's at fault but that this unfairness shouldn't occur. Especially when I've tried to be a responsible person."

"Is It Right to Benefit From AIDS?"

SHAWN

Shawn said his "full-time work" was being a college student. In addition, he volunteered as an AIDS educator. He described conflict about whether he should benefit from having AIDS. "Is it right to use AIDS for my benefit with professors?" Shawn asked. "AIDS puts a lot of stress on me, stress that other students don't have. Since I have the added stress of AIDS, is it right to ask professors for special privileges because of AIDS? Is it right to accept honorariums for speaking about AIDS? Is it right to be paid for the book that I am writing about AIDS?"

Describing his resolution to his conflict, Shawn said, "I think that it is right to use AIDS for my benefit as long as I make some good out of a bad situation. I have started to take advantage of the lenient treatment professors give me because of AIDS. I would like to get honorariums for speaking about AIDS. I hope to make money from the book that I am writing."

"I can justify getting good out of AIDS," Shawn rationalized, "as long as my primary motivation is to help people. Even though I feel bad about taking advantage of professors' leniency toward me because of AIDS, I think that I've got enough bad breaks, and I deserve to be able to take advantage of good breaks when I can."

"Since I have legitimate things to say about AIDS," Shawn went on, "being paid for speaking about AIDS is a legitimate way to support myself. I am writing a book so that people can understand how I feel, and they can better understand AIDS. My only motivation isn't to make money."

"Although I Value the Expertise of Lawyers, Should I Follow Their Advice When I Don't Trust Them?"

DOUGLAS

Douglas, a PWA and "educator," said that because of AIDS, he was experiencing legal problems. He described conflict about the right way to deal with them. Concerned about confidentiality, he did not provide details.

"How can I be sure that I have a lawyer who understands HIV so I get good legal advice?" Douglas asked. "Like living wills, financial situations, and medical situations. Knowing how to go about doing the right thing. If you own a house, a car, insurance. With AIDS, there may be prejudice, and I won't have the same rights I would otherwise. What legally can I do about that? How should I pay for it?"

"When situations arise," Douglas said about his resolution, "I want to go about them in a positive and good way to get the resources that I need. Fortunately, I haven't had to deal with a lot of legal issues yet. The AIDS Project has some person you can consult with about a legal issue."

"Legally," Douglas reasoned, "I think there needs to be more people that can understand and educate. I don't know how much the legal profession knows about AIDS. It's important for legal people to understand how AIDS affects one, one's family. It is important for one with HIV to know that the legal person is educated and unprejudiced."

"Should I Plan a Funeral I Can't Afford or Be Satisfied With a County-Paid Funeral?"

PATRICIA

Patricia, a PWA and "minister," described conflict about whether to plan the kind of funeral that she wanted or be satisfied with a county-paid funeral. "I am on welfare, and the county will bury you. I don't think they take care of the total bill. I don't want to be cremated. I don't want to be buried in a box. I want to be buried in a coffin. I want a funeral. I think three thousand will give you a good funeral."

"What do I do to pay for my funeral?" Patricia asked. "I don't have the money. My children don't have it. How should I make sure that my kids don't have to worry about burying their mother because she did not face the fact that she was going to die and made no arrangements to get resources to bury her? But where do you start? So many resources, you can get lost."

"I'm going to look into how to pay for my funeral," Patricia resolved. "I don't know where I'm going to get the money, but I need to go as far as I can to deal with it. I want to have a good, peaceful death. I want to know that there aren't unfinished things about my death."

Explaining her rationale, Patricia said, "Once you deal with a situation, it's out of the way so it don't keep coming back up. Give you inward peace, and you are relieved of stress. Peace is being able to lay down in my bed, close my eyes and go to sleep without thinking. Not worrying about whether my babies are going to be hungry but having assurance that they're going to eat. It's like cruising and not feeling one bump. Being HIV-positive makes you deal with things where maybe you would have pushed it in your subconscious mind. A lot of foolishness, I don't have time for. I'm more of a fighter now and more aggressive."

Commentary

Some PWAs were poor and discussed long-standing financial problems. As Peggy put it, "You don't make it if you work or don't work." To obtain funds, they were "on welfare," which they said was insufficient for their needs. Catherine said, "After paying my rent, I don't have enough left for the month."

Their stories illustrate financial difficulties facing poor, chronically ill people. "They're putting you in this miserable state, and you have no reason to live," said Catherine. Unless PWAs are critically ill, they may not qualify for some government programs. The sicker they are, the more likely they are to receive government help (Vladeck, 1989).

Other PWAs described financial problems that had arisen because of AIDS and were taking away their middle-class life-styles. Steve, Lisa, and Scott said that they wanted jobs, but working full time endangered their health. As Steve put it, "Either I have to work full time, which physically I can't do, or be totally disabled in order to pay my bills."

On the other hand, they hesitated to stop working. "I liked having the money," said Lisa. "It provided me with insurance. Staying at work provided me with something to do and a good way of self-esteem." Scott said, "Without a job, I feel like a non-person, and I'm lonely."

They wondered if they should try to make ends meet by making themselves eligible for government assistance. However, relying on the government would lead to other ethical problems. "To be disabled," explained Steve, "you have to give up your assets, and you end up in poverty."

Because Scott did not have a job, he could not afford his middle-class apartment. He, like other PWAs documented in the literature (Mandelker, 1987), was experiencing difficulty finding a place to live. "My disability is about to run out," he said, "and I'm worried about ending up on the streets. How could this happen to a guy who had a good job and education?"

The stories of Shawn and Douglas illustrate problems that PWAs from middle-class backgrounds may face although they work full time. Shawn questioned if he should benefit from AIDS. Douglas, like many other PWAs, wondered how to obtain affordable and knowledgeable legal help (Fox, 1987).

The PWAs said that they did not have sufficient information to resolve their ethical problems effectively. "But where do you start?" asked Patricia. "So many resources, you can get lost." Steve said, "They give me one number to call, and they can only talk about one thing. They send me someplace else."

To resolve their conflict, most PWAs no longer worked full time, and they lived on limited income. As Steve put it, "I went bankrupt, got rid of any assets, and only work so much in order to maintain my disability benefits." Some PWAs were considering or were engaging in illegal activities. Peggy said, "I want to go steal," and Steve said, "I don't report most of my income."

The PWAs' stories suggest societal strategies for resolving the kinds of ethical problems described in this chapter. One strategy is to provide job training and jobs that are flexible, full time, and part time. "If there was any fairness," said Scott, "people would be able to get training to work, not necessarily in their field." As Steve said, "I don't see how it is cost-effective if you don't allow people to actualize their potential and give them resources to get back on their feet."

Jobs provide success, self-worth, money, and other benefits that may prolong PWAs' health and ability to remain at home (B. Rogers, 1989). Otherwise, PWAs may need expensive institutionalization, paid for by society (Anderson, 1990). To be effective, these jobs could not jeopardize PWAs' health or the health of workers who are in contact with PWAs (Carrick, 1989).

Another societal strategy is to broaden and coordinate services for PWAs, such as financial assistance, subsidized housing, and legal help (Chang et al., 1992). Describing current services, Steve said, "The disability system is an ethical nightmare, which I hate." If services are coordinated, PWAs will not have to deal with numerous agencies. Service providers need training so they do not aggravate PWAs' ethical problems but help to resolve them (Fox & Thomas, 1990; Vladeck, 1989). PWAs need to be told about available services in language that they can understand. As Steve put it, "There should be informational seminars about available services to teach people how to use the services they're getting."

Finally, the kinds of ethical problems described by the participants can more easily be resolved if individuals in society develop a compassionate attitude toward PWAs. Scott told how his perception had changed. "Now I view people begging for money in a different way. You don't know what they have been through. They don't have anybody to love them."

Of course, society cannot resolve all of the ethical problems addressed in this chapter. PWAs will need to do their part by acting responsibly and working together with society to develop effective resolutions. Douglas described what he was doing. "When situations arise," he said, "I want to go about them in a positive and good way to get the resources that I need." Patricia planned to take positive action so she did not leave unresolved issues for her children after she died. Shawn and Steve expressed interest in benefiting other people.

Whatever the causes, the PWAs faced serious ethical problems involving finances and business. They were desperately dependent on government assistance, in the absence of family support. From their perspective, society should increase their entitlements. With limited resources, society cannot provide entitlements for everyone who requests them. A major ethical problem is: What is the right way to spend public funds? An analysis of society's values is needed to develop effective resolutions.

One model for analyzing society's values is the "New Ethic" research project of the Center for Biomedical Ethics at the University of Minnesota. Project members identified the current values framework and then developed a values framework for health system reform. The consensus was that values should be placed at the forefront of health care reform because we as a society will more likely agree on strategies to resolve the health care system's fundamental problems once we agree on the values that should drive the system (Priester, 1992).

Besides health care, all areas in which public funds are used need to be addressed in order to develop a values framework for guiding expenditures. Various questions need answers: What are society's values? Are they ethically justified? What values would be more ethical? How should public funds be spent in line with society's best values?

If effective resolutions are not quickly developed to the kinds of ethical problems described in this chapter, some PWAs in all likelihood will lead duplicitous lives and engage in crime to deal with intolerable situations. As Peggy put it, "If I get desperate for money or ill so I'm going to die pretty soon, the fear of jail ain't going to stop me." Crime committed by disenfranchised members of society could be much more costly than the expense of efforts to decrease it.

In summary, an ethical society provides an environment in which its members can meet their financial needs. As Scott explained, "I was taught by my parents that you pull your own weight. Contributing is all I know. I'm not supposed to depend on somebody. I'm supposed to help other people. It's not that somebody's at fault, but that this unfairness shouldn't occur. Especially when I've tried to be a responsible person."

9

Ethical Problems Involving Health Care

Do nurses, physicians, dentists, and other health care personnel have an ethical duty to provide care for all persons who come to them? What an astonishing question! Not since the great plagues of earlier centuries has this ethical problem been debated with such fervor. Now questioning is again occurring in relation to PWAs (C. Levine, 1991).

Since HIV disease was first identified, many health care personnel have provided outstanding care for PWAs. They have gone out of their way to make up for society's rejection of PWAs. However, other health care personnel have been reluctant and even unwilling to treat PWAs, despite being given information about AIDS (Ackerman, 1990; Gallop, Lancee, Taerk, Coates, & Fanning, 1992; Jecker, 1990).

For several reasons, health care personnel may hesitate to treat PWAs. Foremost, they may fear becoming HIV-infected themselves (Brennan, 1989; Meisenhelder, 1991). They may disapprove of homosexuality and intravenous drug use, and they may feel discomfort being around dying young people (Alexander & Fitzpatrick, 1991; Gee, 1989; Schwarz, 1989). Finally, they may feel anxious about caring for persons who are culturally dissimilar from them (Fox, Aiken, & Messikomer, 1990).

The fears of health care personnel can aggravate and even create ethical problems for PWAs. Those persons who hesitate to treat PWAs may not provide good care for them. Their discomfort may influence their decisions about allocation of health care resources, such as choosing between multiple competing claims for admission to a limited number of intensive care beds (Levin, Driscoll, & Fleischman, 1991; Zoloth-Dorfman & Carney, 1991).

Nine PWAs (two women and seven men) and a mother of a PWA specifically described ethical problems involving health care: "Should I give up or fight to graduate from a nursing school that rejected me because of being HIV-infected?" "Although I value the expertise of health care personnel, should I follow their advice when I don't trust them?" "Although I value the expertise of health care personnel, should I follow their advice when they don't care about me?" "Although I value the expertise of health care personnel, should I follow their advice that's unwise?" "Although I value the medical expertise of my son's doctor, should I get another doctor who has a heart?"

"Should I Give Up or Fight to Graduate From a Nursing School That Rejected Me Because of Being HIV-Infected?"

KARL

Karl, a PWA with "chronic fatigue, thrush, diarrhea, and night sweats," described conflict about how to deal with a nursing school that rejected him for being HIV-infected. He did not know if he should continue trying to complete the program.

"I'm a licensed practical nurse," Karl began, "and I went into the registered nurse mobility track at a college nursing school. My second year, I was required to be immunized for rubella before my Peds/OB (pediatric/obstetric) rotation. I had ARC (AIDS-related complex), and my immune system was compromised. I refused take the rubella vaccination because it's a live virus, and I didn't want to jeopardize my health."

"I told the director of nursing in confidence that I had ARC," Karl said. "Even though I said I would do all the infection control measures, the nursing school would not let me graduate. They blamed the clinical institution. I wondered if I should fight the system, obtain a false rubella titer, or find another way around this situation."

Describing his resolution, Karl said, "I chose to maintain my integrity by fighting the system. I talked to the clinical institution, and they said that was the Department of Health policy, and AIDS was not the issue. The Department of Health said, 'Each institution sets their standards.' The League for Nursing said, 'We have no governing power over that.' I asked if they would write a restricted license from pediatrics and OB, and they said, 'Sure, as long as you graduate from an accredited nursing school.' So back to square one. I talked with an attorney at the Center for Constitutional Rights in New York. They had difficulty getting information from the school, and they got no response from the League for Nursing."

"After I was diagnosed with AIDS," Karl went on, "I couldn't fight this battle anymore. I didn't have energy or resources. I let go. Now I try to educate people about the broader ethical problems involving AIDS. I addressed the State Senate about discrimination. I spoke to the League for Nursing. I do education for community colleges, nursing programs, and chemical dependency programs and talk about the right thing to do. I say, 'If you are uncomfortable with AIDS care, don't do it. Other people are comfortable and can do that.' "

"Giving up was a big loss," Karl said, explaining his rationale for his resolution. "It was unjust because I had no choice. If I were that director of nursing, I would have called for development of an HIV policy regarding nursing students. I would have gotten together with administration, the legal department of the school, department of health, other schools who have worked out this dilemma, and the League for Nursing."

"A nursing school should let a student who has AIDS or is HIV-positive graduate," Karl continued. "To single out HIV as a reason for excluding somebody is wrong. Somebody who is HIV-positive isn't of danger because it's standard to use universal precautions. I wonder how many nursing students are HIV-positive. When I did a pediatric and obstetrics clinical rotation in LPN [licensed practical nurse] school, I was not required to show a rubella titer, and it was only a year earlier."

"I understand an administrator's fear of being liable," Karl said, "but I fear that policies are made to reduce liability as opposed to being effective. A nursing student who is pregnant may not be able to do all the work that someone who isn't pregnant can do. She shouldn't be prevented from finishing nursing school. The ethical question is fairness to people with disabilities. The law says that educational institutions are not allowed to discriminate on the basis of physical disability."

"If we want to hold professionals accountable for making ethical decisions," Karl concluded, "that should be addressed in education and on licensing exams. Giving professionals ethical problem-solving skills would be more valuable than spending quarters trying to discern what is the difference between hypothecary, metric, and household medication systems. The examples often used are obsolete ethical situations. We need to take a systemic look at nursing."

"Although I Value the Expertise of Health Care Personnel, Should I Follow Their Advice When I Don't Trust Them?"

BRUCE

Bruce, a PWA whose health was "fair/good," said that because he valued the expertise of health care personnel, he participated in research to test AIDS drugs. However, he described conflict about whether to trust his physicians enough to take these drugs.

"I hesitate taking them because I don't know if they do me any good," Bruce said, "and I wonder if they may hurt me. They are unpleasant and inconvenient. When depressed, I don't want to take them and be reminded of AIDS. I want to live a normal life. Not taking them helps me to deny that I have AIDS. When I don't take my medications regularly, I have extra ones at home. Is it right not to take medication that is available to me because I participate in research and not available to other people who want it but don't participate?"

"I go for awhile and take my medicine and then go for awhile and not take it," said Bruce about his resolution to his conflict. "If I'm too busy, I don't take it. If I'm depressed, I don't take it because I want to deny that I have AIDS. I don't participate in drug research that involves a placebo because I want to know what I'm taking."

"I don't take my medicine as often as my doctors want me to take it," Bruce reasoned. "My doctors know that I don't take it regularly, but they don't know the true extent of me not taking it. I haven't drawn any strong conclusions about the benefit of the medicine or I'd probably take it all the time."

NANCY

Nancy, a PWA, described her health as "exhausted." Although she, like Bruce, said that she valued the expertise of health care personnel, she felt conflict about whether to follow their advice when she did not trust them.

"The most conflict I have is with prescriptions," Nancy said. "I want to take them because I don't want to die. When I take the prescriptions, they make me sick because they're toxic. I'm afraid they're hurting me and may make me die faster. I don't know which decision to make."

"I don't know if doctors and nurses take AIDS as serious as I do because it has nothing to do with them," Nancy continued. "My mom's a nurse, and she acts like she has no feeling. Her best friend just died of cancer. They were both RNs. It's just something's going to happen, and you're going to die anyway. Doctors and nurses don't treat me like a human being. I'm a thing, a statistic you study. Sometimes, I think they're trying to take our money. Medicine is so expensive, it's ridiculous. I can't see how somebody could be cold and watch people die because of their studies. Some doctors and nurses are prejudiced because a lot of people with AIDS are drug addicts or gay. Sometimes the drug addicts act like assholes. So doctors and nurses think that everybody with AIDS is the same, and it's not true."

"Confidential things aren't really confidential," Nancy went on. "I feel like they're going to collect us with AIDS some day and do something. They have our information on computers. All this confidential stuff is bullshit because they got writing or a law on the side that can change the confidential paper. Sometimes I feel like this was a germ warfare."

"Doctors and nurses can't do anything for me, so why should I do what they want?" asked Nancy. "All they do is take blood so they can study. I can't stand needles, and I don't want them taking my blood. Nothing ever happens. It costs all this money for them to tell me that. I don't know if I'll die quicker by doing what they want or by not doing what they want. I don't know what is the right thing to do."

Nancy described her resolution to her conflict. "Sometimes I take the medication," she said, "and sometimes I don't. That's screwing me up. I told the doctors I wasn't going to take it anymore. They put me on another medication and said they'd check my blood count again. They'll watch it more closer with me."

Explaining her rationale to her resolution, Nancy said, "I don't want to die. I lack information about my disease. The doctors have the information, but they don't tell me. I would like to be more involved in the study about it. I come up with ideas and wonder if they would work. They could have a hospital especially for AIDS. That way the patients could be more involved, working with the scientists that are studying it."

BILL

Bill, a PWA who described his health as "stable," commented, "Medication helps me because it slows down the process but doesn't help me because it makes me miserable. Should I take it anyway and hopefully prolong my life? Medication killed someone I know. If the doctor would have made sure the patient understood, he might be in pain, but he'd be living. I believe there is a cure, but they aren't telling us because of money."

"How should I deal with medical staff who talk in technical terms?" Bill asked. "They say, I told him that he was going to die. But it's disinformation because they told you, but they didn't tell you. They use technical terms to protect themselves because they don't want to deal with harsh realities. The medical establishment is definitely an obstacle for ethnic groups. The Third World is not represented in teaching hospitals. All these people are from Japan and Korea. Their English is terrible. So they don't convey the information to the patient like they should."

"How should I deal with medical staff whose main concern is money and prestige?" Bill asked. "When they have no other means of evading a question, they say it costs money. They don't care. It's just a job. I work with people that I wouldn't be seen with. But I do it because it pays well. These doctors are the same. The more patients, the more money and grants you get from the government. They take your money and treat you any way they want."

"I see a doctor but don't take medications," Bill resolved. "They take my blood and see if there's any dramatic changes. I try not to get stressed out about the medical establishment. I say, 'Bring me information so I can understand why I'm sick and what to do about it. Don't tell me to take five pills every day and everything is going to be fine. I'm not going to listen to you because I don't believe a word you say.' "

"I don't take medications because they don't work for me," Bill reasoned. "I've come to serenity in myself. This is my personal idea of saving my life. I know my body better than medical staff because I'm the one that takes the medication. Until doctors and staff break language down where everyday people can comprehend what they're saying, I don't think that person should take medication because he doesn't know what the doctor's telling him."

"I can't go around dwelling about when I'm going to die," concluded Bill, "but I want to make it as far away as possible. I want to feel good and be out of stressful situations. That's what life is about, and it took AIDS to explain it to me. It would take stress off if they had ethnic doctors and nurses."

GARY

"I am angry at doctors," Gary, another PWA who described his health as "stable," said. "When I found out about having HIV, my wife was pregnant. They were scaring her that our son would come out with AIDS. I said, 'You don't be telling her that. When my son is born, we'll see what goes on.' He was born. He was tested. He's 100% negative. He's going to be a big, healthy boy."

"Why give me medicine now that's been out for 5 years?" Gary asked. "I should have started before. All they say is they don't know why. 'It is up to me if I want to take chances with side effects.' I say, 'Fine. I haven't had side effects.' Can I trust what they're saying? Is it working?"

Describing his resolution, Gary said, "I don't keep doctors' appointments, but I take my medicine five times a day. I go for regular blood drawing and to get another prescription."

Gary reasoned, "My doctors let me know what's going on. That's how I think it should be. My mother don't understand why I don't keep doctors' appointments. A doctor cannot tell me what I already know. I don't want to sit there so you can poke on me, because there's no need to. Why go to the doctor if they're not going to do some good for me? All they do is sit and talk."

"Although I Value the Expertise of Health Care Personnel, Should I Follow Their Advice When They Don't Care About Me?"

BARB

Barb, a PWA, told me that she was troubled with "thyroid and low blood." She said that although she valued the expertise of health care personnel, she felt conflict concerning whether to follow their advice when she did not think that they cared about her.

"I don't think doctors and nurses care," Barb said. "They brush you off like a cold potato, especially if you are on medical assistance.

It's wrong that they don't take your word and check it out thoroughly. By the time they try to correct what's wrong, be too late. When I say something's wrong, it's wrong. If you pay, they will listen. They get paid, and we ain't getting paid for going to them. You feel alone because the doctor doesn't want to listen. Who is there that cares?"

"I don't know if I trust the doctor to tell me the truth," Barb continued. "What caused AIDS? Needles, blood transfusions, sex? They're not telling the truth about it. I was doing drugs, and then I wasn't. I was having sex with different people, and then I wasn't. Why don't none of my kids have it? It's a puzzle that can't be put together."

Barb resolved, "I'm not going to the doctor anymore. Why tell them about it? Ain't give you nothing."

Explaining her rationale, Barb said, "I think the doctors should take more responsibilities in their job. They should believe the patients. Listen to how you feel. They say, we don't know, and then they want you to talk to other people."

NEAL

Neal, a PWA, said that because his mouth was infected by "thrush," he had difficulty eating, and he was trying to gain back the 10 pounds he had lost. Although he, like Barb, explained that he valued the expertise of health care personnel, he described conflict about the right way to deal with those whom he did not perceive as caring about him.

"One week," Neal began, "the physician that followed me was off. I was seen by his partner who said, 'There's nothing in your chart about your last visit.' That's irresponsible. I contemplated suicide. I wasn't getting good medical care."

"I still experience health care workers that are fearful of giving me hugs or eating with me or holding my hand or kissing me on the cheek," Neal continued. "They can't deliver good comprehensive care. Their fear tends to make them angry, and they want to protect themselves."

Neal described his resolution to his conflict. "I've become an AIDS activist and make presentations about AIDS," he said. "My goal is for people not to go through what I'm going through, because it's miserable. Hopefully, I can remove the fear and hysteria that people have about those afflicted with HIV."

"Physicians should feel their patients are important enough to do good documentation in their charts," said Neal, explaining his rationale. "Physicians have about 15 minutes for a patient. That's not enough time to do good management. Prior to a patient being seen, clinics could go over the chart. Were tests done and the results given to the patient? Was the person referred to other physicians, and were they talking with the referring physician? If not, follow through. They should look after the patient like managing anything."

"Who is going to help if the doctors can't?" asked Neal. "Emotional support gives you that added incentive to keep on, especially with the knowledge there is no cure. Your life is tenuous, especially when there's a constant opportunistic infection going. It makes everyday living a little trying."

"I care because I've always loved people," said Neal. "I would not wish this disease on anyone. If I can keep someone from having this virus transmitted to them, I've succeeded. I think my presentations ease people's fears. When they don't fear, they can give good comprehensive care in a caring way that comes from their heart versus from fear. That's better care than if they focus on medical sorts of things."

ROY

Roy, a PWA, told me about "severe pain" and a "rash all over my body" that kept him from sleeping. He questioned how to deal with health care personnel whom he did not think cared about him.

"A nurse mix my medication, and I don't know what I was taking and didn't like it," Roy began. "When I'm hurting, and I call them up and tell them what's wrong, they can never get a hold of the doctor. I need help and won't call because they tell me a lie.

I stubborn, especially if I think you're doing me wrong. There's nobody I could call if I get sick. I live by myself and lonely."

"My doctor is power-hungry," Roy said. "She not interested in what's wrong with me. They don't like Blacks. The student doctors are redneck, too. I know because of the way they treat you. Even the girls that setting to the desk don't like Blacks. They put you down. They act like they scared of me because I got AIDS. That bother me. I said, 'Hey, man, why in the hell you won't get another job? Then you don't got to deal with AIDS people.' One reason, I don't know how many Blacks go the clinic. White people got AIDS, they don't act like they're scared of them."

"Let me tell you how the nurses treat me," Roy continued. "They got a smoking lounge in the hospital. I go in there and watch TV to keep from laying in bed all day because bed ain't good for me. If I'm there and you know where I'm at, why go in my room and set my pills in there and don't tell me? The nurses take my food and do the same thing. Walking to my room is further than walking to where I was."

Describing his resolution to his conflict, Roy said, "That why, cut me loose. I don't let myself be abused. I don't want to go to my doctor and complain. I just curse them out and go about my business. Now I have a doctor that I like."

"I believe my doctor's doing everything he can to help me," Roy reasoned. "I don't like people. I likes to be alone. I don't like to see any human being get abused. I been abused. I watched my sister and mother get abused. I wanted to kill myself because I didn't like the world, because of what happened to me. It's rough, it's really rough. To have AIDS and be Black."

"Although I Value the Expertise of Health Care Personnel, Should I Follow Their Advice That's Unwise?"

DAVID

Like the PWAs described above, David said that he valued the expertise of health care personnel, but he described conflict about whether he should follow their advice that was unwise. He did not explain the situation because of confidentiality. "The medical profession is concerned," David said. "Unfortunately, it's different, living with AIDS, opposed to treating it. I don't think they realize how that can affect one. They know this is their duty, and they're going to try to do the best that they can." David explained that in trying to be helpful, his physician sometimes gave him legal advice. "I recently took some information to my physician regarding my illness and was not informed properly to comfortably feel that I was doing the right thing," he said. He felt pressure to follow his physician's advice, which might not be wise advice and could lead to serious consequences.

Although David was not sure how to resolve his conflict, he was leaning away from taking his physician's advice, reasoning, "I don't want to worry that when I give this information, what kind of consequences I might suffer. I don't think they are educated enough in the legal area to advise. A legal issue for someone who is not infected might be different than for someone who is. I don't know if they realize the difference. Sometimes that can cause confusion. The medical profession can give advice to a certain extent, but not about legal things."

"Although I Value the Medical Expertise of My Son's Doctor, Should I Get Another Doctor Who Has a Heart?"

SUE

Sue, a significant person, said that she valued the expertise of health care personnel. However, she was unhappy with the physician of her son, a PWA, and she questioned if she should get another physician for him.

"I don't like him," Sue said about her son's physician. "He's good medically, but he lacks integrity. He's judgmental, punitive, belittling, and doesn't communicate with the family. He's prejudiced toward my son, who hasn't used drugs in years. 'Can't be a good person if you are a drug addict,' [he thinks]."

"When my son made a joke about the medicine," said Sue, "the doctor said, 'You've gotten good medical care, and if you keep this bad attitude, I'm going to send you to another hospital.' My son said to him, 'I'll take the medication.' I just sat there and gritted my jaw and said to myself, 'Don't do anything that's going to jeopardize his medical care.' "

"The doctor told my son to take a medication twice a day," Sue continued. "The doctor should have clearly communicated that to me. I did not tell the doctor that my son forgot to take two more packages. He'd just yell at me. So I gave my son the other two on Saturday and Sunday, which should have been double-dosed on Thursday and Friday."

"I talked to the nurse who calls periodically to find out how my son is doing because she cares," Sue went on. "She said this doctor had a mind-set and to find another doctor. I don't know if I should stay with the doctor or get another one. This decision is difficult because the medical care he gets with the hospital staff is superb. I'm afraid if we get another doctor, we will be put out of the hospital. The doctor is the medical director there. My other son says, 'Shine him on. He only does the prescribing. We don't need any comfort from him. We get it from the people who actually give the hands-on care.' "

"It's tough because my son doesn't have a doctor that I feel is a friend," Sue said, "somebody that I can work together with in partnership. That gives him a lot of power over our life, which is frustrating, putting it mildly. I have confidence in his medical abilities. His ability to communicate as a human being is not good, and that might jeopardize my son's treatment."

Sue described her resolution to her conflict. "Right now," she said, "I'm trying to shine him on. I'm looking into getting another doctor and going to the same hospital."

In regard to her rationale for her resolution, Sue explained, "It's very important that doctors care. There's not much else they can do. At least give the families a little comfort. They need it. I need someone to give me a tap on the shoulder and say, 'It's OK.' Loving, caring is what makes life bearable. Without caring, life looks bleak, and then why keep on living? Might as well be a piece of machinery and not a human. If the heart is missing, one is not really a human being."

"This doctor seems to be missing a heart for my son, for me, for my family," Sue concluded. "Some patients care for him, so I'm sure it's there somewhere. The doctor not only should be astute medically, but be compassionate, communicative. A doctor should have integrity. When you take the oath, you're supposed to put prejudice aside but, being human, that doesn't always happen. That's what I mean by that he's lacking integrity."

Commentary

The PWAs and a mother of a PWA described ethical problems that they said resulted from disrespectful, untrustworthy, uncaring, and unwise health care personnel. Although they perceived some health care personnel as treating them well, they felt alienated from and distrustful of others. Their stories illustrate paternalism, stigmatization, classism, and racism in the health care system, and they suggest how health care personnel can treat each other with dignity and provide better care for clients.

Karl's ethical problem could become increasingly common as more health care personnel, like other members of society, are diagnosed with HIV disease. When an undergraduate nursing program did not allow Karl to graduate because of being HIV-infected, Karl said that the health care personnel whom he contacted to ask for help did not treat him respectfully. "The ethical question is fairness to people with disabilities," said Karl. "Institutions should not discriminate because of HIV."

Of the 25 PWAs, 7 told me that they had been or were health care personnel, although 4 of these persons had retired because of deteriorating health. Although 6 PWAs said that they had become HIV-infected away from the job, one PWA may have been exposed to HIV disease as a result of a needle stick on the job. This PWA had engaged in unprotected sex off the job, which also may have been a mode of exposure to the disease.

Surprisingly, Karl was the only PWA to discuss an ethical problem regarding discrimination toward HIV-infected health care personnel. Three PWAs, described in Chapter 12, talked about how having AIDS was affecting their work. They described conflict concerning the right way to balance their needs with the needs of their clients in order to avoid jeopardizing their health. However, they did not address other ethical problems on the job because of their HIV status.

Moreover, none of these health care personnel brought up ethical problems involving HIV transmission to their clients. They did not say if they told their clients or employers about having AIDS themselves. Even a PWA who worked as a nurse in hemodialysis, which is a high-risk area for needle sticks, did not discuss the possibility of infecting clients or other employees, other than to mention the importance of universal precautions.

The health care personnel with AIDS seemed more concerned about their own personal problems than client-related problems. Perhaps they carefully used universal precautions on the job. However, not all other HIV-infected health care personnel may be as cautious. Additional research is needed to learn more about the extent to which HIV-infected health care personnel avoid infecting clients and other employees.

To resolve ethical problems involving HIV-infected health care personnel, health care organizations are developing policies regarding how HIV-infected health care personnel should conduct their work (American Nurses Association, 1992). These policies need to protect clients, while respecting the confidentiality and livelihood of health care personnel (Adler, 1991; Daniels, 1991; Lo & Steinbrook, 1992; Lovejoy, 1991; New York Academy of Medicine, 1991). Otherwise, such policies could have the reverse effect of what is intended by actually discouraging health care personnel from being tested for HIV and limiting their practice in ways that reduce the risk of HIV transmission (Nelson, 1991).

Ethical policies need to address circumstances under which HIV-infected health care personnel should be restricted from providing client care and doing invasive procedures (Glover & Starkeson, 1989; Smith, Stevenson, Keeling, & Herrick, 1989). These policies need to be based on thoughtful, ethical analysis and facts about HIV transmission, rather than stereotypes and fear. They need to include careful monitoring and counseling of HIV-infected health care personnel in an atmosphere of trust, privacy, nondiscrimination, and support (Schulman, 1992).

Finally, ethical policies about HIV-infected health care personnel need to enhance clients' trust. Scientists see the risk of clients contracting HIV disease from health care personnel as an exceedingly rare event that is costly to prevent (Danila et al., 1991). Ethicists have argued that given the minimal risk, mandatory testing of health care personnel would not be cost-effective (Coulter, 1991; Daniels, 1992; Glantz, Mariner, & Annas, 1992).

Clients, on the other hand, see the risk as a personally dreadful event. Without knowing the HIV status of health care personnel, they would be taking this risk involuntarily (Blendon et al., 1992). The public demand for mandatory testing of health care personnel and penalties for concealment of positive test results needs to be addressed in a calm manner in order to encourage public trust (Lo & Steinbrook, 1992).

The stories told by Bruce, Nancy, Bill, and Gary illustrate why some clients may distrust health care personnel. For one thing, these PWAs did not believe that health care personnel always had their best interests at heart. As Nancy put it, "I'm a thing, a statistic you study."

Like other PWAs, these PWAs took part in research to assure easy access to expensive, investigational medications (Ackiron, 1991; Edgar & Rothman, 1990; Freedman & McGill/Boston Research Group, 1989; Schulman, Lynn, Glick, & Eisenberg, 1991). However, they seldom took their medications, which could adversely affect their health and the research results. Questions arise about whether consent to participate in such research is fully informed, especially for women and people of color (Murphy, 1991d; Schulman, 1992; Sorrell, 1991). To avoid these problems, research needs to be structured to protect clients and produce accurate results (Arras, 1990; Pierce & VanDeVeer, 1988).

Another reason for mistrust was that Bruce, Nancy, Bill, and Gary thought that some health care personnel cared more for money and prestige than treating them. "Medicine is so expensive, it's ridiculous," said Nancy. Bill commented, "I believe there is a cure, but they aren't telling us because of money. They take your money and treat you any way they want."

Health care is costly, particularly for PWAs, and often it revolves around health care personnel, not clients (Bennett, Pascal, & Cvitanic, 1992). To reduce these problems, many health care organizations, including the nursing profession, have supported a national health care system that focuses on wellness and care instead of illness and cure. Ideally, this new system would assure access, quality, and services at affordable prices. Each client would receive a basic core of essential services that are offered at familiar sites, such as schools, workplaces, and homes. Rather than being structured for the convenience of health care personnel, the new health care system would adapt to the needs of clients (American Nurses Association, 1991).

A third reason that Bruce, Nancy, Bill, and Gary distrusted some health care personnel was because they feared that their confidentiality was not being protected. As Nancy put it, "Confidential things aren't really confidential." Although state health departments have taken steps to ensure security of HIV data (Torres, Turner, Harkness, & Istre, 1991), the participants' fears may be realistic. Unfortunately, some health care personnel may justify breaching PWAs' confidentiality on the grounds of a duty to warn others about AIDS (Fleck, 1991).

A fourth reason was because of cultural insensitivity by some health care personnel. "The medical establishment is definitely an obstacle for ethnic groups," explained Bill. "They use technical terms to protect themselves because they don't want to deal with harsh realities. It's disinformation because they told you but didn't tell you."

Bill suggested how this mistrust could be decreased. "It would take stress off if they had ethnic doctors and nurses," he explained. Nancy offered another suggestion, "They could have a hospital especially for AIDS. That way the patients could be more involved, working with the scientists that are studying it." Nursing and medical schools have begun to address this mistrust by offering more content about cultural diversity.

The stories told by Barb, Neal, Roy, and Sue illustrate uncaring health care personnel. As Barb put it, "They brush you off like a cold potato, especially if you are on medical assistance." Neal said, "I still experience health care workers that are fearful of me." Roy commented, "It's rough, it's really rough. To have AIDS and be Black." Sue explained, "My son's doctor is good medically, but he lacks integrity. This doctor seems to be missing a heart."

Neal and Sue talked about why health care personnel need to show caring for their clients. As Neal explained, "Emotional support gives you that added incentive to keep on, especially with the knowledge there is no cure." Sue said, "It's very important that doctors care. There's not much else they can do."

Although some health care personnel described by the PWAs may never have been caring persons, others may have lost their ability to care. Perhaps they felt stress because of constraints within the system, anger from clients about their deteriorating health, and unresolved grief concerning clients who died (Stein, Wade, & Smith, 1991). Their resulting diminished sense of self-esteem and ethical responsibility may have caused them to shift their focus from clients to themselves and climbing the career ladder (May, 1992; Quill, 1991; Schwarz, 1989; Zuger, 1991).

The participants suggested how health care personnel can be more caring. Barb said that doctors should "listen to how you feel." Neal recommended, "Physicians should feel their patients are important enough to do good documentation in their charts. Prior to a patient being seen, clinics could go over the chart. They should look after the patient like managing anything."

Of course, the primary way that health care personnel can care for persons with HIV disease is by treating them without prejudice. Ethicists have argued that health care personnel consent to a standard level of risk of infection when they enter the field and, in most instances, the risk of contracting HIV infection does not exceed this level (Daniels, 1991). Professional organizations have published codes of ethics and positions papers that describe health care personnel's ethical mandate to provide care to clients who need it, regardless of their social and economic status or personal attributes (American Nurses Association, 1985, 1992; Goldman & Stryker, 1991; National League for Nursing, 1988). However, many nurses, physicians, dentists, and other health care personnel have hesitated and even refused to care for persons with HIV disease (Pierce & VanDeVeer, 1988; Wiley, Heath, Acklin, Earl, & Barnard, 1990). For the most part, they are afraid of the health risk that they face from occupational exposure to HIV disease. In particular, persons who work in an emergency room, surgical suite, hemodialysis center, or intensive care unit may be in danger because they routinely handle blood products and needles that could infect them (Raviglione et al., 1992).

The risks of occupational exposure to HIV infection can be reduced or eliminated as health care agencies institute engineering controls. Another way is by mandating the use of universal precautions for handling blood and body fluids (Department of Labor, 1989). To diminish the fear of occupational transmission, policies are being developed that provide some protection for health care personnel (American Nurses Association, 1992; Brennan, 1991).

Research indicates that health care personnel's fear of persons with HIV disease may be due in part to misinformation (Campbell et al., 1991; Ficarrotto, Grade, & Zegans, 1991). The fears of some health care personnel decreased when they were given accurate information (Armstrong-Esther & Hewitt, 1990; Brown et al., 1990; Swanson et al., 1990). Education can help health care personnel to provide quality care for persons with HIV disease, while taking precautions to avoid becoming HIV-infected themselves (Gemson et al., 1991; Husted & Husted, 1991; Jemmott, Jemmott, & Cruz-Collins, 1992; McNabb & Keller, 1991; Purdon, 1992).

Karl suggested that health care personnel need to learn about ethics as well as HIV disease. "If we want to hold professionals accountable for making ethical decisions," he said, "that should be addressed in education and on licensing exams." Including ethics content could help health care personnel to develop critical thinking and give better client care (Lewis & Eakes, 1992). Moreover, ethics education for health care personnel could stimulate development of effective resolutions to ethical problems involving homosexuality, drug abuse, confidentiality, treatment options, refusal of treatment, routine testing of clients, and death and dying (Downes, 1991; Grady, 1992; Hitchcock & Wilson, 1992; Lewis & Coffee, 1991; Lombardo et al., 1991; Macklin, 1991; Manzella, Falk, McConville, & Kellogg, 1992; Rothman & Tynan, 1990). Educators could help health care personnel to debate the right way to balance their conflicting values about clients, science, their profession, institutions, society, and themselves (Nelkin, Willis, & Parris, 1990; Webb & Bunting, 1992).

Not only would providing education about HIV disease and ethics lead to quality care for clients, but such education would in all likelihood reduce the occurrence of ethical problems like the one described by David. His story illustrates the importance of health care personnel giving wise advice, rather than venturing into areas such as legal issues about which they are not qualified, even though they may have good intentions.

Health care personnel by themselves cannot resolve all ethical problems related to the health care system. PWAs need to do their part, too. The participants explained how they were dealing with their ethical problems. Bruce, Nancy, Bill, Gary, and David carefully determined when to follow the advice of health care personnel. Barb and Roy avoided health care personnel whom they perceived to be uncaring, whereas Sue was dealing with her son's physician by "trying to shine him on."

Karl and Neal became AIDS activists in order to teach health care personnel about AIDS and ethics. As Neal put it, "When they don't fear, they can give good comprehensive care in a caring way that comes from their heart versus from fear. That's better care than if they focus on medical sorts of things."

In summary, the lover of a PWA suggested what health care personnel can do about the kinds of ethical problems discussed in this chapter. "Give clients written instructions about medications and treatments," he said. "Follow through on what they request. Treat them as human beings and peers. Listen to what they say to know if their needs are being met. Be their advocates. Realize how vulnerable and powerless bedridden people are. Explain what will be done before doing it, not afterward. Let them know that they won't be penalized for complaining about poor care. Do treatments and medications the way they are supposed to be done, rather than in a haphazard or inaccurate way."

10

Ethical Problems Involving Personhood

Persons with AIDS (PWAs) face rejection by their families and society, deteriorating health and finances, and premature death. Like other people in similar situations, they may question who they are and what values will help them to deal with their changing circumstances. Various studies indicate a high level of depression, anxiety, panic, and suicidal tendencies among PWAs. Although some PWAs may feel hopeless, other PWAs are turning their experience into an opportunity for personal growth (Adair, Nygard, Maddox, & Adair, 1991; Barrows & Halgin, 1988).

Among the major mysteries still surrounding AIDS is why some people live in vigorous health for years after being diagnosed with HIV disease, while others become ill and die (Pfeiffer, 1992). At present, treatment for HIV disease provided through the health care system consists primarily of combating the virus and secondary infections. Another treatment is to enhance immune system functioning. Although medications and other therapies have not yet been developed to strengthen immune operation, behavioral strategies may help persons with HIV infection to be long-term survivors (Adair et al., 1991).

The participants said that their attitudes affected their health. They questioned what kind of values they should hold in order to feel good about themselves and enhance their health or the health of their loved one with AIDS. To develop effective answers to this question, they were grappling with their beliefs about God and religion, as illustrated in Figure 10.1.

The longer an interview went on, the more the person's ethical conflict centered on personhood. In fact, 13 PWAs (1 woman and 12 men) and four significant persons (two women and two men) specifically described ethical problems involving personhood: "Should I believe in God and religion even though I have problems with them?" "Should I be who I am or somebody else?" "Should I be a good person or a bad person?" "Should I keep going or give up?" "Should I be accepting or angry?" "Should I admit my powerlessness or try to control everything?"

"Should I Believe in God and Religion Even Though I Have Problems With Them?"

JAKE

Jake, a PWA in his forties, said that he was "strongly spiritual but not religious." He described conflict about whether to believe in God and religion.

"Should I be a Catholic?" Jake asked. "As a small child I had sexual feelings that were different than other people's feelings. Because the Catholic Church rejects gay people, I developed self-hatred. I can't reject everything because the Catholic Church is too much a part of my history. I need to develop my spirituality in order to recover from alcoholism and drug abuse and to cope with AIDS. How can I nurture my spirituality while rejecting the destructive aspects of the Catholic Church?"

Describing his resolution to his conflict, Jake said, "Through AIDS I realize that my spirituality is separate from being Catholic. I've given my life to my inner power and have been guided, loved, and nurtured ever since. When a Catholic tells me that I am a sinner, I tell the person that I do not feel that way. The Catholic

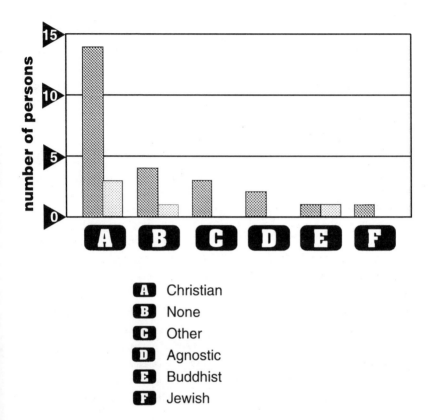

Figure 10.1. Self-Reported Descriptions of 25 Persons With AIDS (PWAs) and 5 Significant Persons (SPs) About Their Religion

Church can't hurt me if I'm not willing to let it. I acknowledge that I am a Catholic and show love to Catholics."

"Knowing that I am not the only person struggling with these issues helps me," said Jake. "I have become part of a growing, nurturing support network of persons who are from a variety of backgrounds like Catholic, Episcopalian, Lutheran, and Jewish. We share our spirituality with each other."

Jake explained his rationale for his resolution. "Spirituality is different from religion," he said. "Being spiritual means realizing that I have an inner power which guides me and holds the mysteries of wonder, life, and change. I can be spiritual and pray without going to church and subscribing to dogma. It doesn't make any difference what the men in Rome say about my sexuality. God does not hate me or see me as an evil person. I know that my sexuality is blessed by God. All of us, regardless of our beliefs, share spirituality and inner energy."

FRED

Fred, a PWA in his twenties, said that he was an "agnostic," although he had been raised as a Christian. Like Jake, Fred described conflict about whether to believe in God and religion.

"If there is a God," Fred asked, "why do I have AIDS, and why is there so much bad in the world? God sure doesn't have control over anything, or how could God let bad go on? Since God doesn't do anything about the bad, there must not be a God. Should I believe in God in order to have the comfort of knowing that I will go to heaven when I die?"

"Even though I call myself an agnostic," Fred said, describing his resolution, "I may have some beliefs about God and religion because they affect my view of right and wrong. I don't know if there is a God. I don't necessarily believe that there's going to be an afterlife or heaven or hell."

"Something had to happen to spark life on the planet," Fred reasoned. "Whatever sparked life doesn't have supernatural powers and doesn't have control over things. It would be comforting to have solid religious beliefs in God and heaven, but I can only go as it comes."

PAULA

Paula, a significant person in her twenties, said that she was Fred's girlfriend and had been raised a Christian. "I don't go to church anymore," she began, "and I don't know what to believe about life after death. One belief sounds good one week, and another belief sounds good another week. I don't want to worry about this when I am young. It is more scary not to know what happens after death than to know that there is nothing. You can't be optimistic if you know that nothing happens after death or something bad takes place. It seems like something pleasant should happen after death to give purpose to life."

Describing her resolution, Paula said, "Since I don't know what happens after death, for me the purpose in life is to do what is morally right, which also helps me. What's morally right is to help other people first. I want to act in such a way that I am not in conflict with myself. I don't want to be selfish, putting my feelings first, but putting other people in front."

"If something happens after death," Paula reasoned, "the best way to prepare is do what is morally right. Then I will go to heaven if there is a heaven. What I think is right may not be what other people think is right. Deep down, I think something good happens after death. It would still pay to do what is morally right even if there is no reward after death. I'd be happy and know that I did what I was supposed to do, what fit my internal values."

"Should I Be Who I Am or Somebody Else?"

EDMUND

Although he had been brought up Catholic, Edmund, a PWA in his twenties, said he was a "nondenominational Christian." He described conflict about whether to be himself or someone else.

"I was fighting who I am," he said. "I never realized where I fit in. I've had the impostors' disease. But I could never be good enough. If I couldn't be those things, who was I? If my identity was based on what other people wanted and they abandoned me, I wouldn't have my identity at all. That was the ultimate fear for me. Do I exist if I'm not defined?"

"I am enough," Edmund resolved. "I have to be OK with me. I'm starting to see self-esteem I never had. I'm learning a different way of grounding. I read meditation books, pray, and try to be honest with people. I try to get my needs met in a healthy way that says that I care about myself. I'm getting what I need from people. They support and reinforce what I'm doing."

"I'm a child of God," he reasoned, "worthy of all the universe has to offer. If you're a cow, you're a cow. If you're you, you're you. As I am true to myself, I'm becoming all that I wanted to be. What makes life worth living is a sense of self, of belonging. Hearing kids play, waking up without a hangover, not wondering if the person I had sex with last night is going to get HIV, being humble. Humility is not thinking of yourself as less, but thinking less of yourself. Now I don't think of myself as the big guy or drug dealer. I'm a part of everything."

"Should I Be a Good Person or a Bad Person?"

RICHARD

Richard, a PWA, was in his thirties. He said that he now considered himself to be "agnostic," although he had been raised as a Christian. He described conflict about what kind of a person to be: Should he be a good person or a bad person?

"How can the world have an ethical order when I've tried to be a good person, and yet I have AIDS?" Richard asked. "Does it pay to be a good person? I don't know if I'll wake up with another physical problem, or how long I have to live. How should I behave when I don't know what is going to happen next?"

"I am trying to be a good person," Richard resolved, "loving, caring, hospitable, independent, honest, hardworking, self-sufficient. I want quality in my life. I have become less materialistic, because it doesn't matter how much money I make or what type of clothes I wear. I will work to make a living, but it's not as important now. It's more important that I have good friendships and improve my relationships."

Richard explained his rationale for his resolution. "I have learned to trust people more," he said. "What is important is to live as long as I can and, in the process, contribute to other people's lives in terms of their own happiness or their ability to help me, which is important to some people."

JACK

Jack, Richard's lover and a significant person, was in his thirties. He said that he did not have a religion, but he described conflict about whether to be a good person or bad one. "Should I remain fully in my relationship?" asked Jack. "Sometimes running away or taking my life seems preferable to dealing with the pain of loving someone with AIDS. Should I continue in my monogamous relationship and be frustrated, or meet my sexual needs with someone else? My lover isn't interested in sex because of AIDS, and we haven't had sex for a year. How should I show affection to him and protect myself from HIV? Even though I rationally know how HIV is transmitted, I worry that he might infect me when I kiss him."

"Should I let my lover deal with the health care system on his own and take the risk that things won't go well, or be his advocate?" he asked. "As a patient, he is vulnerable to nurses and doctors who don't treat him as a human being. He doesn't always obtain all the information he needs about medications and treatments. If I take on the role of advocate, I will need to learn what I can and deal directly with the nurses and doctors on his behalf."

"For now," Jack resolved, "I will remain in the relationship and structure my life so that things move along in a peaceful, steady fashion. Even though I've been looking around, I want to remain monogamous. I avoid becoming infected. I will try to be his advocate by listening to the nurses and doctors to learn about medications and treatments. I will encourage them to treat him like a human being and follow through on what they say. I will ask them for what he needs when he can't ask them."

Jack reasoned, "I love him too much to not be fully in the relationship. Most of the time, staying monogamous feels like the right decision. Sex isn't a need that has to be met right now. If I engage in right thinking, I won't be infected when he and I are careful. If I am his advocate, he will get better health care, and things will go more smoothly."

MIKE

Mike, a PWA in his twenties, said that he was raised a Christian but now did not have a religion. He, too, described conflict about whether to be a good person or a bad person.

"I want to please myself and other people," Mike said, "but often our needs conflict. How can I feel good about myself, and have others feel good about me, too, especially if I die soon?

"I want to be polite, willing to help people when there's nothing in it for me but the satisfaction of helping them, and have a good relationship with my family. I'm more selfish than I'd like to be. Selfish means being greedy, primarily concerned with myself and what's going to give me immediate happiness."

"To feel good about myself," Mike said about his resolution, "I try to be a nice person who is unselfish. I've developed a closer relationship with my family."

Mike reasoned, "I should be a nice person in order to feel good about myself, rather than to please God or the church. It's important to be nice to people because you never know how many chances you are going to have to make impressions on people. There's no reason to be a total jerk to anyone. The important thing is on your death bed to feel good about your life. You'll feel better about your life if you've been a nice, good person."

HARRIET

Harriet, Mike's girlfriend and a significant person, was in her twenties. Raised a Lutheran, she described conflict about whether to be a good person or a bad person.

"Should I blame gays for my boyfriend having AIDS?" Harriet asked. "He does, and so does my support group. Should I blame God? I was raised Lutheran, but I don't go to church. I wonder if religion could give me some comfort in dealing with AIDS. How can I resolve the issues about AIDS so that I will feel happy and

everyone else will, too? It's an unattainable goal. I'm a perfection-
ist and want to do everything right."

Describing her resolution to her conflict, Harriet said, "I don't
blame AIDS on gays or anyone else. I don't blame God for AIDS
since it's just luck what happens. I can't control luck so I let go. I
don't go to church, because religion isn't such a good deal for me
anymore. I know that I can't resolve issues about AIDS in a way
that will make me and everyone else happy. My fear of rejection
has mellowed since I was a child."

"You can't blame AIDS on anyone because no one knew how it
is transmitted," Harriet reasoned. "It's not good that my boyfriend
blames gays for AIDS, but at least he doesn't blame AIDS on
himself. Blaming God for AIDS is a cop out. Life isn't fair. Bad
things just happen. I don't think it would do much good to be
angry at God because you can't touch or see God. You can get mad
at the church, but what good does that do?"

"Should I Keep Going or Give Up?"

GLEN

When I asked Glen, a PWA in his forties, about his religion, he
replied, "No particular dogma." He, too, was concerned about
personhood and described conflict about whether to keep going
or give up.

"When I was diagnosed," Glen said, "I felt overwhelmed, threatened, scared. I could give up, believe that I would die in a month.
Should I confront AIDS, as I previously had with alcohol and drugs?
I knew from Alcoholics Anonymous that by being honest about
AIDS, I would live more fully than denying it, and I would
continue on my wonderful, spiritual, healing journey. If I didn't,
I would give AIDS more power than it had, like I gave to alcohol
and drugs. I knew I wouldn't have to face AIDS alone because I
could ask for help."

"I embraced AIDS and called out for help," Glen said about his
resolution. "My experience with recovery from alcoholism and

drug use served as a foundation. AIDS is part of life, not my whole life. I take good care of my body. I don't view HIV in a hostile way. I love it, more as how can we beat this together? I meditate and go to my healing circle. I give speeches, appear on television, and write articles to share spiritual energy. Being on my spiritual, healing journey resolves many ethical problems for me. I don't have many ethical problems because they resolve themselves."

Glen explained his rationale for his resolution. "It's a mystery why I decided to become sober and start on this spiritual journey," he said. "By confronting my fears, they don't have me. My confidence and self-respect have grown considerably. When I realized that I could call for help and help was there, it taught me that I could be there for other people, that caring and nurturing each other is part of our humanity. If you love yourself, you're capable of loving another. The love you give is the love you get. I'm grateful to AIDS for opening my sense of empowerment. AIDS is a gift."

DONALD

Donald, a PWA in his forties, was a "Roman Catholic" who like Glen described conflict about whether to give up or keep going. "I want to say, screw it," Donald began, "and then I think, 'I've got a good chance of being alive, so keep going.' So we don't give up, should my wife and I participate in support groups? We're not interested in groups where you get a bunch of woe-is-me people talking about their problems. I want support that will help me to keep going and be a asset, not a burden to my family or society—to deal with my anger about the scientific community's slow response to AIDS."

"I keep going," Donald resolved. "I try not to hurt anybody, and if I can do something good for someone, I do it. I try to live by the Golden Rule, treat people as you want them to treat you. We have not gotten into support groups because they don't treat me as a normal person. I stopped asking, 'Why me, God?' I would be willing to work on AIDS education and discrimination as long as they wouldn't know that I have AIDS. It's something I ought to do."

"Why stop now because I have AIDS?" Donald asked, explaining his rationale. "There ain't no justice or AIDS would not happen. I can control my little section of the world by being a good person. If I treat other people correctly, they're more likely to treat me correctly. If everyone does that, it will all help. Most of the time I am a good person and live up to my values."

"God is responsible for HIV," Donald said, "but he's also responsible for me living this long. So it's a balancing-off thing. If I get to meet him, I'll say, 'What the hell does all of this mean?' Tune in a million years from now to see if there is some good coming from HIV."

Should I Be Accepting or Angry?

LLOYD

Explaining that he did not have a religion, Lloyd, a PWA in his fifties, described conflict about whether to be accepting of or angry about AIDS. "One part of me isn't worried about HIV," he said, "but another part is. At time, I feel like nothing going to happen. I got poisoned with shooting speed. 'I've made it through other tough things, so I'll make it through this one, too.' That's not what my mind is saying, but deep down I'm pretty sure that's what it is. It doesn't frighten me."

Describing his resolution, Lloyd said, "When I feel angry about AIDS and start thinking about death, I always go down here to the store and get me a half a pint of strong whisky, and I sit in there, and drink, and go ahead and go to bed. I don't get up 'till the next morning. HIV is something that I got, and I accept it. I go to see the doctor and nurse regularly."

"Never had no conflict about the right thing to do," Lloyd reasoned. "My mind be clear when I drink, like hatred going out of me. HIV doesn't affect me that much because I'm not afraid of dying. My doctor and nurse was honest with me, and I believed them. The doctor said, 'You in good health. That's why I'm not giving you no medicine.' The nurse told me if I used drugs, 'Make sure no one ever used them and they're clean.' She explained different ways to have sex. I feel good about how they've treated me. I don't think they treat me differently because of being Black."

BENJAMIN

Like Lloyd, Benjamin, a PWA in his twenties who said that he did not have a religion, described conflict about whether to be accepting of or angry about AIDS. "It gets to me sometimes," he said. "Make me feel angry at the world. I can't stop taking my medicine, but it hard to take. What worries me most is that I will get sick. The death part doesn't fear me. That's the part of AIDS I don't think about."

"I live day by day," Benjamin resolved, "being careful to a certain extent. I've slowed down a lot because my bones have got older. I'm still active. I still shoot basketball, ride bikes, go jogging, and try to keep my body in good shape. I know AIDS is there. If I do get sick, I probably won't worry about it. But I'll know I have it."

Explaining his rationale, Benjamin said, "I'm not going to let AIDS ruin my life. If I do, I might as well die instead of messing up everybody else's life. I got a will for wanting to stay here until the good Lord feel it's time for me to go. I enjoy living. I think that's why I lived this long. The good thing about living is fresh air, sunlight, being around people I love. I don't want to miss nothing. The best thing is watching everything change. My main reason for wanting to live is to see my son grow up. He will be able to live a full healthy life and do things that I wanted to do and couldn't."

JOANNE

A "Protestant" PWA in her sixties, Joanne described conflict about whether to be accepting of or angry about AIDS. "We've led a healthy life," she said, "been monogamous, haven't used IV drugs, and yet I have AIDS. How should I live with this unfairness, this death sentence? How can the world have order when I've obeyed the rules and yet been punished with AIDS? AIDS is not a pleasant death. You are pressured into doing all the things you wanted to do. My husband and kids don't like to lose their mother. It's a hopeless feeling for everybody when they hear it. They don't know what to say."

"I don't know that we've resolved accepting AIDS," Joanne said about her resolution. "I've tried to have a positive attitude and keep fighting, appreciate each day. My husband has been a big support. We go to the HIV clinic and a support group, and we went abroad. We don't postpone things. I'm not so fussy about cleaning. When something stresses me, we try to resolve it. We invested in insurance so that we'd have something left for my husband and kids. We've been honest with people about AIDS. We've have spoken to groups to educate them, and we have been in the papers."

Joanne rationalized, "Going to the HIV clinic and telling people gives us the feeling that we are doing something positive, which gives hope and is therapy. We're not hiding. Telling people is the right thing to do because we have a good understanding of AIDS. People have been wonderful, good acceptance. I don't think they are going to come through with a cure fast enough for me. Sometimes I feel better that it's me rather than younger people. It's God's doing that I've felt great. I feel like I'm going to be around for quite awhile. I have a lot of things to do yet."

RON

Ron, a significant person and Joanne's husband, was "Protestant" and in his sixties. He, too, described conflict about whether to be accepting of AIDS. "Why us?" he asked. "The irrationality is hard to accept. The reality of losing my wife is constantly with me. Some days I feel I will be able to handle it, and other days it's rough. You would like to pull the shades down, lock the door, sit there, and feel sorry for yourself, or deny things, be a butterfly, and shoot the works."

Ron described his resolution. "You cling to what is true and real," he said, "what you live by, who you are. These solid values became important, values of family, friendships, faith in God, love for each other. We let slide other things such as social living, money, entertainment. We decided that life is worth living. You stay with it and try to move ahead. We are trying to get a balance of responsible living while enjoying what time we have together.

We know there will be tough times ahead. If we keep up our hope, we will cope with them."

"Sometimes people tell jokes that are hard to handle," Ron said. "We keep in mind that people are people. We participate in research and stay abreast of the latest happenings. We pray for the Lord's hand to be on the researchers. We told our kids, other relatives, neighbors. Now we are talking to groups. We have been on the radio and television and in the papers. We are involved with a huge support group because of all the people we have talked to."

"Why us? It's happenstance," he reasoned. "You take the good with the bad. If you don't accept, you have a problem. Struggling with adversity is part of growing. The middle of the road is right for us. To determine the right way, we bounce our ideas back and forth. We don't usually come up with an answer right away. Helping other people is good therapy. If we can help one person, it will be worth it. We enjoy trying to educate people. They open their arms to us in compassionate love. We are satisfied with what we've done with our lives. We have a good family, and we've done the things we've wanted to do. We've been successful in our careers. What else can you ask for?"

"Should I Admit My Powerlessness or Try to Control Everything?"

RUSS

Describing his religion as "various," Russ, a PWA in his forties, questioned if he should admit his powerlessness or try to control everything. "Society portrays people who are HIV-infected by a blood transfusion as poor, unfortunate victims and gays and IV drug users as bringing AIDS upon themselves," he said. "Since I'm gay, how should I deal with this perception?"

"I can't control society," resolved Russ, "but I can see all of us with AIDS as participants, not victims." He reasoned, "I didn't bring AIDS upon myself. I don't want to have AIDS. I didn't have sex because I thought I could have AIDS. Because I participated in life, I'm a participant like persons who have become infected with HIV through blood transfusions."

TIM

Like Russ, Tim, a PWA in his forties with "no particular religion," described conflict about whether to admit his powerlessness or try to control everything. "As a man," he began, "I think I should be in control, but I feel out of control because of AIDS. Men have been controlling and powerful for a long time, and if I'm a man I should be, too. I also feel out of control because I am gay. I am confronted with rejection by male-dominated controllers who say that I am less than manly. I feel sad about things over which I have no control."

Describing his resolution to his conflict, Tim said, "I've had to give up controlling. I accept that I'm a man, even though I'm not in control, and generally I like that I'm a man. I accept that I'm a gay man. I accept that I don't have the secrets of all these wonderful mysteries. I don't get caught up in wishing anymore. I don't cry over spilt milk."

"The more I give up control and open myself," Tim reasoned, "the more empowered I feel, and the more successful I am at sharing my inner power and at gaining energy and spiritual power from other people. We create an energy flow that is strong, positive, and growing. This has affected my immune system in a positive, nurturing way, and I feel good, fulfilled, and blessed. There are things in my life that I'm grateful for not having any control of. Wishes are a trap. Often they are tied to materialism, which can be destructive. If I don't wish, I accept what the world, the moment, holds for me. Accepting my powerlessness is more gratifying and spiritually edifying. AIDS has been the key that opened the door to the lessons I've learned."

MARK

Mark, a Lutheran PWA in his twenties, described conflict about whether to admit his powerlessness or try to control everything.

"I would like to deny having AIDS in order to believe that I am in control," he said, "but that doesn't work. AIDS takes away physical health. The only thing left is my mental health and that feels out of control, too. I've blown up for the dumbest reasons. I need counseling to relieve the stress, but I can't call a counselor because I see that as being out of control. I consider that I'm failing as a human being because I need somebody else to heal my mind."

"I've started to accept that I have AIDS, and to treat it like terminal cancer or some blood disease," Mark said about his resolution to his conflict. "I no longer treat it like lepers in the Bible. I've got the name and number of a counselor. Now I've got to break down and call this person."

"Because AIDS is becoming more socially acceptable," Mark reasoned, "other people are accepting me, and I'm accepting myself more. I can't do anything about having AIDS, so I might as well accept it. I think that it would be good for me to accept having AIDS and calling a counselor."

Commentary

The participants' ethical problems involving personhood illustrate the interconnectedness of ethics and theology, the study of God/higher power (Aristotle, 1987; Flaskerud, 1992; Fortunato, 1987; Frankena, 1973; Noddings, 1984). In part, the participants were asking age-old theological questions that confront each person: Why me, God? How can the world have an ethical order when I've tried to be a good person, and yet I have AIDS (or another problem)? How should I live and die when I do not know if an ethical order exists or what happens after death?

Some PWAs found help in organized religion. For PWAs who had experienced difficulties with organized religion, however, these questions were particularly difficult to answer. Fred said that even though he had been raised a "Christian," he was now an "agnostic" and did not go to church anymore. "It would be comforting to have solid religious beliefs in God and heaven," he said, "but I can only go as it comes." Jake talked about nurturing his spirituality while rejecting destructive aspects of organized religion, and Russ struggled to develop spirituality in spite of society's perceptions of gay men who become HIV-infected as bringing the disease on themselves.

Like the PWAs, the significant persons who had experienced difficulties with organized religion said that these questions were difficult to answer. "Should I blame God for my boyfriend having AIDS?" asked Harriet. "I don't go to church anymore, and I don't know what to believe about life after death."

With the exception of Lloyd, all of the participants talked about their struggle to develop answers that would help them to make some sense of their suffering and live as well and as long as possible. Generally, they tried to answer the first question (Why me, God?) with a kind of acceptance. "I can't do anything about having AIDS," explained Mark, "so I might as well accept it." Donald said, "I stopped asking, 'Why me, God?' "

In various ways, the participants answered the second question (How can the world have an ethical order when I've tried to be a good person, and yet I have AIDS or my loved one has AIDS?). "God is responsible for HIV, but he's also responsible for me living this long," said Donald. "There ain't no justice or AIDS would not happen." Harriet explained, "I don't blame God for AIDS since it's just luck what happens."

The third question (How should I live and die when I do not know if an ethical order exists or what happens after death?) was related to the participants' desire for meaning. They wondered if life without an ethical order had purpose, and a purposeless life seemed bleak. Their answer was to be virtuous, whether or not an ethical order exists. "I should be a nice person in order to feel good about myself," said Mike, "rather than to please God or the church." Paula reasoned, "Since I don't know what happens after death, for me the purpose in life is to do what is morally right. I'd be happy and know that I did what I was supposed to do, what fit my internal values."

For participants who had experienced difficulties with organized religion, viewing spirituality as being different from religion helped them to develop answers to these questions. As Jake put it,

"Being spiritual means realizing that I have an inner power which guides me and holds the mysteries of wonder, life, and change. I can be spiritual and pray without going to church and subscribing to dogma." These participants described spirituality as harmony with the whole of things, which many of them called God. For them, spirituality was closely related to meaning and integrity. They defined *meaning* as seeing one's life as being part of a bigger, purposeful picture and *integrity* as living in harmony with one's values. In contrast, *religion* referred to sectarian dogma, which they associated with unsympathetic organizations.

The discovery of theological concerns in the participants' ethical problems is not surprising. From the beginning of time, human beings have wondered whether ethical living depends on theological beliefs (Benjamin & Curtis, 1992; Frankena, 1973). Analyzing the relationship between ethics and theology is beyond the scope of this book. However, the participants' stories illustrate the importance of acknowledging theological aspects of ethical problems. Unless these concerns are directly addressed, individuals who are experiencing ethical problems may not be able to develop effective resolutions.

Ethical listening, described in Chapter 15, is a strategy for facilitating individuals' discussion of their ethical problems, including theological concerns. By listening ethically, a person may be able to help someone to resolve an ethical problem effectively. I used ethical listening to help the participants to describe their ethical problems. All of them thanked me for listening to them. Over and over, they wished for a nonjudgmental person to confide in about what was bothering them. I wondered how their ethical conflict was affecting their immune function and whether effectively resolving this conflict would enhance their health and perhaps even help them to live longer.

Recent research indicates that deep, unresolved conflict can affect the immune system. The experience of long-term survivors may provide new hope and direction for persons with HIV disease. Over several years, researchers have carefully examined physical, psychological, and spiritual factors that may strengthen or jeopardize immune system functioning. The findings suggest that behavior strategies may help HIV-infected persons to be long-term survivors (Adair et al., 1991; Pfeiffer, 1992). Adair et al. (1991) reported that long-term AIDS survivors cared for their physical health through moderate exercise, a nutritious diet, sufficient rest, and systematic relaxation. By developing positive attitudes and reducing their fear, anxiety, anger, and hostility, they took into account their psychological health. They met their spiritual needs by being joyful and engaging in the three kinds of love: sexual love, friendship, and love of God/higher power.

Furthermore, long-term survivors with AIDS tended to have helpful contact with another PWA, and they participated in a support group. Feeling some control over their lives, they took responsibility for their health and believed that they could influence the outcome. They did not take a passive, compliant role or a defiant, adversarial role with health care personnel. Instead, they worked in partnership with them. Altruistically involved with other people, they had a sense of purpose in life (Adair et al., 1991).

The participants' stories support this research. "The more I give up control and open myself," said Tim, "the more empowered I feel, and the more successful I am at sharing my inner power and at gaining energy and spiritual power from other people. This has affected my immune system in a positive, nurturing way."

Their stories illustrate the need for support services that enhance the immune system function of persons with HIV disease. Such services would provide people who listen ethically and help clients to resolve their ethical problems, including theological concerns. Because many persons with HIV disease feel profoundly distrustful of authority, especially religious authority, these services need to be carefully planned and administered, and confidentiality needs to be an important part (Macklin, 1991).

In some areas of the United States, walk-in peer counseling centers are being developed for persons with HIV disease (Levinson & Miller, 1992). Some religious organizations are throwing open their doors. Support groups are being set up in hospitals and other agencies (Buck, 1991; Kendall, 1992). Unfortunately, these services may be more focused on crisis intervention than the kinds of philosophical and theological questions that the participants were trying to answer.

To be effective, providers of support services need education in AIDS and ethics (Knox & Gaies, 1992) so that they can skillfully engage in ethical listening. They need to develop understanding of HIV-infected persons' experience, rather than impose their own values (Nokes & Carver, 1991). Then they will be more likely to help persons with HIV disease resolve their ethical problems in a manner that leads to meaning, integrity, and longer, more satisfying lives.

In summary, the participants not only talked about their struggles, but they also shared what they had gained from their ethical problems involving personhood. Glen, Jake, and Edmund had raised their self-esteem, and Richard and Glen had developed better relationships. In the process of educating other people about AIDS, Joanne and her husband, Ron, had been helped themselves. Amazingly, Glen and Tim expressed appreciation. As Glen put it, "I'm grateful to AIDS for opening my sense of empowerment. AIDS is a gift." Tim explained, "AIDS has been the key that opened the door to the lessons I've learned."

11

Ethical Problems Involving Relationships

AIDS poses a threat to PWAs' relationships. Dealing with AIDS in a traditional relationship with social support, such as heterosexual marriage, is difficult in the best of circumstances. In nontraditional relationships with little or no social support, the stress can be even greater (van den Boom, 1991). Besides worrying about HIV transmission, many PWAs and their loved ones face multiple losses and cumulative grief from death due to AIDS of partners, parents, children, and friends, and they struggle to balance emotional engagement and detachment (Carmack, 1992).

Of particular concern are relationships among parents and children. Most women and children with HIV disease are urban, poor people of color (Capell et al., 1992). The cities in which they reside face serious economic problems that contribute to family and social disintegration (Heagarty & Abrams, 1992). Questions arise about the right way to keep parents from transmitting HIV disease to their children, who should take care of children whose HIV-infected parents cannot provide for them, what should be done about children who are HIV-infected, and who should pay for and provide their care (Boland & Conviser, 1992; Enfantis, 1991; Faden, Geller, & Powers, 1991; Stuber, 1992).

Although HIV infection in America has been a disease of homosexual and drug-using men, increasingly women and children are becoming infected. Attention to the disease in women and children lags behind attention given to men (Heagarty & Abrams, 1992). This chapter addresses ethical problems resulting from HIV disease in women and children and ethical problems involving relationships that are seldom addressed in the literature.

Figure 11.1 illustrates the relationship status of the 30 participants. Eleven PWAs and 3 significant persons said that they had children. Fourteen PWAs (7 women and 7 men) and 2 significant persons (1 man and 1 woman) specifically described ethical problems involving relationships: "Should I have a child even though I have AIDS?" "How should I balance my needs with the needs of my child?" "How should I balance my needs with the needs of my partner?" "How should I balance my needs with the needs of my family and friends?"

"Should I Have a Child Even Though I Have AIDS?"

ROGER

Roger, a PWA who was gay and did not have any children, wondered whether he should have a child. "What troubles me most," he said, "is not being able to procreate, wanting to see yourself in someone else. Choosing to be gay, I realized I wasn't going to have a child. I grieve over not being able to have children. If I'd held true and gotten married to the girl I was in love with and had a child, maybe I would never have contracted HIV. Or maybe it wouldn't have happened until after I had a child. Should I make a woman pregnant in order to have a child? I've always been attracted to women. But I can't imagine a woman responsibly taking on that burden to perhaps infect herself with HIV. I could try without being responsible."

"Ethically, that's not where I am today, to be irresponsible sexually," Roger resolved. "I could not bring myself to be that selfish, have that lack of concern for another human life. So I share

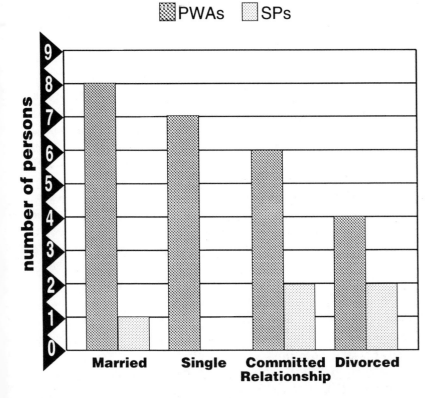

Figure 11.1. Self-Reported Descriptions of 25 Persons With AIDS (PWAs) and 5 Significant Persons (SPs) About Their Relationship Status

where I can. I love children. I work with kids from all age groups as an AIDS educator. I look at their faces, the glow, radiance, and all the things that children have, the innocence."

"I would not want a child to come into this world having to deal with HIV," he reasoned. "Abusive behavior—drugs, sex, rock and roll, people—is not an option because it takes away from what I have. I want to make the right choices, be responsible to myself, the universe, sense of spirit, people. Our connection is far greater than we're capable of understanding."

"How Should I Balance My Needs With the Needs of My Child?"

SALLY

For 3 years, Sally, a PWA, had been in a "committed relationship" with a woman, other than when she had injected drugs and engaged in sex with men. Because of drugs, the state had taken away parental rights to her two oldest children. Newly sober, she wanted to keep her newborn, and she described conflict about how to balance her needs with her daughter's needs.

"Should I raise my baby myself or give her to someone to raise?" Sally asked. "They don't know yet if she is HIV-infected. If I get sick and die, she'd be attached to me, and that would hurt her. There's no saying what would happen to her after I'm gone. If I keep her, who will care for her when I get sick? My partner, who also has AIDS, won't be able to take care of her. I don't want my child going to the state, like I did and get stuck in the system. I'd rather have her in a home with a caring family. The shuffle between foster homes is emotionally damaging because you have no sense of family, of belonging."

"It's harder to give her up than my other two children," Sally continued. "I never really had them because I was using drugs. They were taken away from me by the state. I don't want to give her up, but I know I should. It's hard to see my child raised by someone else. I love her and wish I could take care of her, but I can't. Should I keep her for my own needs? Is it less selfish to give her to somebody else so she doesn't have to experience the losses that I experienced?"

Describing her resolution, Sally said, "Right now, I'm planning her adoption. A friend of mine does work with AIDS. She said that she'd be willing to raise my daughter because she had foster children who she's adopted before. I still have visitation rights so I see her when I want to. She'll know that I'm her mom, but she'll always have someone there."

"It's more important to do what's best for her than me," Sally rationalized, "whether I want to or not. It would be selfish of me to keep my baby. This is the way to be a good parent. Ultimately, this is better for me because I don't want to be worrying about her. I'm comfortable with it because I know it's the right decision. I'm OK with the person who's bringing her up. They're doing a good job."

PATSY

Patsy and Conrad, who had AIDS, said that because of their own violence and substance abuse, the state had removed their four minor children from the home. They wondered about the right way to balance their needs and their children's needs.

"I was away from my mom because of her drinking problem," Patsy said. "I don't want that to happen to my kids. Two of them are in foster care, and two are adopted. It's painful that they aren't living with me. I'm afraid if they would find out that I'd died, they'd run away, something bad happen. How should I explain it to them? After I'm gone, I guess it don't matter."

"I've told them a little about AIDS," Patsy said about her resolution, "but I don't want to upset them. I haven't told them that I could die because I don't know. They don't understand. They were checked for HIV and came out OK. I'm happy about that. I try to see them when I can."

Patsy reasoned, "I want to be the one to tell my kids because I'd rather have them hear it from me than someone else. I could probably comfort them more. I don't want them to have to be pushed around like I did."

CONRAD

Describing his conflict, Conrad said, "The state took the kids when they were born because she wasn't capable of taking care of them. When I got out of prison, I brought the kids home. Her and I fight, and she go to a shelter. She go to child protector and sign lies that get the kids out of the home. I was in the work house, took a drink, and didn't go back because they was going to lock me up. The judge held it against me, and I can't see my kids or talk to them on the phone. Now that I have AIDS, it's death coming, and

I want to spend time with my kids. I wasn't in prison for abusing her or the kids. She was in prison for forgery and checks. I want to do right by them, let them know I care more for them more than myself."

"I wonder if I should blow somebody's brains out, child protector, doctor, social workers," Conrad went on. "My wife used to call the social worker twice a week and say she ain't got no food to eat, that I beat her up and took the money. The social worker hate me and bring her money. If we hadn't had kids together I would have left. My wife said people trick my son into saying I had sex with him. He said, 'Mama, Dad ain't did nothing like that.' I was ready to strangle them to death. Hell, I never had sex with my kid."

"I'll talk with the AIDS Educator about getting my kids back," Conrad resolved. "She's going to see if she can't straighten it out. I won't leave my wife." He reasoned, "My kids should be with their father and mother instead of in a foster home. I wouldn't dare leave this woman, which is the best thing I could do. She's completely helpless because when I met her she was some state guardian. They would pay for her rent. Sometime I don't think she know the truth from a lie."

ALICE

Alice, a PWA who was "almost divorced" and had four minor children, said, "When I was little, I was getting in trouble and was adopted. Without blood relatives, what do I do with my kids? How do you tell, 'Kids, I'm dying but I don't know when'? My kids need me, and if I died, they'd go to my half-sister, but she's White and my kids are half-Black and need their culture."

"I got a lawyer through AIDS Foundation to write on paper that my half-sister would take my kids when I'm ready to die," Alice said about her resolution. "I didn't tell them that I had AIDS, except the oldest. I told them, I'm not going to live forever because I'm sick. They understood that."

"I don't know when I'm going to die," Alice reasoned, "so I straightened out what will happen to my kids. I didn't want to tell them I had AIDS because I didn't want them to worry about and have problems in school. There's no good way to tell them without making them feel bad."

JANE

Jane, a PWA, was married with three grown children. "My husband and I wondered if we should tell our kids about my diagnosis," she began, "and if so, when? Reasons not to tell: It hurt me to tell them that I have a horrible disease. I couldn't do anything except get my blood checked. Our daughters were pregnant, and we didn't want to upset them. They would lose their mom, and their kids wouldn't have their gramma."

Jane continued, "Reasons to tell: Eventually, they would have to face it. They have the right to know because they are our kids. We promised to be honest with them. More things would come up, and they would wonder why. I felt pulled between my desire to be honest and my desire to avoid hurting them."

"For 2 years," Jane said about her resolution, "we didn't tell them. We told them when I was in [AIDS] treatment, we were doing something about it and felt more hopeful. My daughters' babies had been born. My husband did the talking. They had a hard time accepting it and went through stages as we did."

Explaining her rationale for her resolution, Jane said, "We weren't dishonest, we were shielding them. The right thing to do is the honest thing to do. If you expect them to be honest with you, you've got to be honest with them. I'm glad about how we told them. It's been easier, and we freely discuss it. They ask questions and feel part of treatment. They are concerned and try to relieve stress. They've been wonderful support."

WES

Wes, a significant person and Jane's husband, described conflict about the right way to balance his needs with the needs of their children. He, too, questioned if and when they should tell their children about her diagnosis.

"At first," Wes said, "there were many reasons not to tell. The hardest part was saying, 'You may lose your mother.' There was misinformation about the disease. We didn't have our feet on the ground. There wasn't anything good to say at that time. We didn't want to tell them when they were pregnant. Later, there were many reasons to tell. We could hold up hope because of medications and research. We'd gone through stages of acceptance and could help them. We wanted them to have time with her before something serious happened."

Wes described his resolution to his conflict. "We told them at Thanksgiving," he said, "in order to give thanks for the hope that we could give them. They went through denial, anger, frustration, shock. We gave them assistance through those phases because we had been through them, too. They forgave us for not being totally honest and made changes so they could be closer to home and see us more often. We became a closer family than normal. We are proud of them."

"You have to face reality and accept things," Wes reasoned. "The kids have a right to know about their mother even though it's not right to hurt them with bad news. The right way is a reasonable way, not doing things in a hurry, keeping your feet on the ground. We told our kids the right way because they were ready, and it worked out well."

BELITA

Belita, a PWA, said that she was divorced with six children, of whom three were grown and three were teenagers. At her home, she held one of her five preschool grandchildren on each knee while the other three sat on chairs next to her. From one child to the next, she put teaspoons of food into their mouths.

"One of my fears is they will take my grandchildren out of my home," Belita said when we were alone. "The kids are placed with me through the courts because of some things with my daughter. My energy is not good. If I could get help, I could keep my kids. But I'm afraid to tell the social worker about AIDS. Will he say I'm not able to take care of them? I don't want my family separated.

Black women used to keeping our families together. Do I have to fight to keep them here? Do I want to fight to keep them here? Should I try to find other resources or go on, and do the best I can?" "I don't know how to deal with this problem," Belita said about her resolution. "I want help from social service so I can keep my kids, but I don't like fighting these people. I want them to treat me with compassion and understanding. I don't want them to keep telling me to try somewhere else."

"A mother live longer," Belita rationalized, "when she can be sick on her sofa and see her baby. That give her energy, not just lay down and die. When you take her children from her, she going to worry about how they doing. Keep my family together would make my health better and my grandchildren happy."

"People know what AIDS is," Belita concluded, "but they need to understand it from the heart. I don't want pity, when they don't treat you like a person anymore. I want your love and compassion. I want you to know me as a human being. We can share some time, and you begin to understand me. A little kid can tell when people really care."

"How Should I Balance My Needs With the Needs of My Partner?"

JASON

Jason, a PWA who was gay and did not have children, described conflict about how to balance his needs with the needs of his partner. "Even though my parents don't want me to tell other members of my family about my being gay and having AIDS," he said, "my lover wants me to tell them. My parents have accepted my lover, but they don't want me to tell the rest of the family about him. I don't want to hurt other members of my family with painful news, but I want them to recognize, particularly if I die, that my lover has been a significant person in my life. By not being honest with them, I obey my parents but treat my lover unfairly."

Jason described his resolution, saying, "Without telling my parents, I may select nonjudgmental persons in my family to tell about my having a gay lover and about AIDS. I will let these people selectively tell other members of my family." Explaining his rationale, he said, "I want to be fair to my lover. He can use the support of my family in times of trouble."

CRAIG

Craig, a PWA who was gay with no children, described a similar problem. "I don't know if I should tell him that I had safe sex one time with another man when I was on a trip," he said. "Fortunately, I knew that I was HIV-positive and told that person before having sex. Since I value monogamy and honesty, I feel guilty and have a sinking feeling in my stomach when I think about it. I want to be honest with him, but if I tell, I risk hurting him and losing his trust in me. I minimize this insignificant sexual encounter because it was safe sex. But he may not minimize it and may think it meant more than it did."

"I am considering telling my partner about this sexual encounter," said Craig about his resolution. "I want to be honest," he explained, "and get this sexual encounter behind us. I think that he would understand."

GINA

Gina, a PWA who did not have children and was in a "committed relationship with a woman," said, "I knew the risk, but blindly went into a relationship with someone who has AIDS. Because our time is limited, I want her to myself, which is selfish, weird. I get strange and don't want to let go. Would it be less painful to leave the relationship or stay in it? Down the road she could die, and I'd be alone. I'll be more attached to her if I stay. I don't want to put someone through a dying situation. Do we want to go through this much pain and turmoil?"

"There's not much time," she resolved, "so I don't go out and do things separately on nights she has off. We don't talk about the death part, the losing each other part. I will never leave the relationship. I wouldn't have a relationship or sleep with somebody who's not infected with HIV. If my partner wasn't around, I wouldn't be involved with anyone. Isn't that weird?"

Explaining her rationale for her resolution, Gina said, "I want to stay in the relationship. I'm so weird, I don't want to spread the virus. There's safe sex, but it's not so safe. I don't put down anybody with HIV for having sex with someone who isn't infected. Whether to have sex is a personal decision."

DOROTHY

Dorothy, a PWA with two grown children from a previous marriage, was now married to a man with AIDS. She questioned the right way to balance her needs with the needs of her husband.

"How should I deal with him?" Dorothy asked. "Before he got sick, he was a healthy, humorous man. Now a world of darkness is there, and you think there is no way out. People get angry when they have a deadly disease. I'm scared he's going to get critically sick again, and he can't do nothing for himself. I'll have to take care of him. It's hard to see somebody you love suffer. I can only do so much."

"The Lord showed me from the Bible how to love and handle my husband," she said of her resolution. " 'If any man lack wisdom, let him ask of God.' Those words gave me strength. I don't think of me, I'm directed towards him. Even though I have AIDS, I do things I love. I encourage him to be positive. Somebody got to bring excitement in the house, and I'm the one to do it. I do my best to make him laugh and let him know life goes on. I have seen changes in his personality. There is inner peace."

"By getting wisdom from God," said Dorothy, explaining her rationale for her resolution, "I have less stress. Daily praying, reading the Bible, going to church. An ill loved one don't need negative things, they need positive. Otherwise, your health will go down when you start worrying, don't have peace of mind, I don't care how much medication you take or if you eat right. I was brought up in the old-fashion way. A husband come first. When you push your problem aside and do something for somebody else, you forget what you're going through. You need that togetherness with your husband. Fear, depression, loneliness destroy. I thank God we have each other."

SAUL

Saul, a single PWA without children, wondered how to balance his needs with the needs of his girlfriend. "Is it right to remain in a relationship with my girlfriend?" he asked. "I love her and want to be sexual with her, but I am concerned that being with me will hurt her. She could get AIDS from me. She could be hurt if I die. My having AIDS brings a lot of stress into her life. I am concerned that because of the stress of AIDS, she might abandon me. Can I help her best, show the most love for her, by staying with her and having sexual relations with her, by just being friends, or by staying out of her life altogether? There's no way for me not to hurt her."

"This ethical problem isn't resolved for me," he said. "Sometimes I think we shouldn't have a relationship. Other times, I think we're doing the right thing to have a relationship. My thoughts change according to circumstances. For now, I will remain in my relationship. We talk about our fears concerning AIDS. She says that she loves me and is willing to accept the risks involved with AIDS. We have a sexual relationship. We use protected sex. I try not to have lots of sexual activity, like on a daily basis. I feel tense and bad about condoms that break and fall off."

Saul reasoned, "We care about each other. Deciding not to have a relationship would be difficult. The alternative is not to have a relationship with anyone I care about. She knows the whole situation and the risks that she's taking. She's in this relationship by choice. Having a relationship with her seems like the right thing to do, because she's happy, and I'm happy, and things have worked out. You never know what is the right thing, but I go by feeling and instinct, my internal values."

HELENE

Helene, a significant person who was "almost engaged" to Saul and did not have children, discussed conflict about the right way to balance her needs with his needs. "Should I stay in a relationship with my boyfriend?" she asked. "By loving a person who may die, am I setting myself up to be abandoned? He may decide that he's too sick and gross-looking to see me. I have a choice about leaving AIDS behind. He doesn't. Since his last girlfriend left, I feel pressure to stay with him and not be like her. I don't want to be hurt by him, but I don't want to hurt him by leaving him. I love him too much to hurt him."

"At night," Helene continued, "I worry about every imaginable thing that could happen, like what if I get AIDS? I would like to marry him and have kids, but I can't until they do something about AIDS. I worry about after he dies, and I find someone else. Will I have to block out his memory? That would be painful. Is it better to leave now and not know what happens to him or to stick with him through the whole thing?"

Helene resolved, "For now, I will stay in my relationship. I take it day-to-day. Things that normally I'd be worried about seem trivial, such as signing eight school forms in triplicate and not knowing where to hand it in. Now I get it done without worrying about it. I don't worry if something has to wait for 2 days. Nobody will die over it. It's more important to do something enjoyable with him, such as bumming around."

Explaining her rationale, Helene said, "I don't know why I love him. Feeling sorry for him doesn't have anything to do with it. I stay because I love him. He's the best guy around, and I couldn't leave him. I cry about losing him, but I can't think of dating anybody else. Part of the purpose of life is to make life better, and we make each other's lives better. He encourages me to get over my shyness, and I help him with a positive attitude."

"How Should I Balance My Needs With the Needs of My Family and Friends?"

TODD

Todd, a PWA who had been in a "monogamous, gay relationship for 9 years," did not have children. He questioned the right way to balance his needs and those of his family and friends.

"How should I tell them that I have AIDS in a manner that will cause them to support me?" Todd asked. "Will I be able to communicate to them my desire for a path of spiritual growth? Otherwise, their fears may overwhelm me and I could become fearful again. They may reject and not help me. How should I deal with their sadness about my AIDS diagnosis? I don't want to cause them pain, but I don't want to get caught in the trap of feeling guilty about causing them pain. Should I support my friends' ways of dealing with AIDS that aren't good for me? Some of them are concerned about confidentiality, which limits their ability to reach out for support. How should I meet my needs without interfering with their meeting their needs?"

"I've been honest with my family and friends about having AIDS," Todd said about his resolution to his conflict. "I try to deal honestly with issues as they arise, and they are generally resolved. I want to be an open, honest person who reaches out for help. I ask for help when I need it, and that establishes a foundation of trust and support that works for me. I resist keeping someone else's confidentiality, especially if I think that the fear of exposure is hurting the person or me. I remind myself that persons have the right to their own opinions, even the ones that differ from mine."

"I am a good friend and supportive person," Todd said. "I continue my healing, spiritual journey. I have learned to like myself, and I'm one of my best friends. I say affirmations in a mirror, a growing experience. I love my family and friends dearly and pray that they will come to the same understanding that I have been blessed with. Through my friendship and care, I may be able to provide for them a key. Instead of letting myself feel guilty about their sadness, I give them love. I realize that people make choices about being sad about AIDS."

"Being honest gives a wonderful feeling," Todd rationalized. "I have a growing, strong ego, and I find strength and support within myself. There are similarities among people, but each person's healing journey is individual. I don't have control over other people. I can't do a great deal about other people's reactions other than to be a caring, loving, supportive person."

NATE

Nate, a PWA, said that he was in a "gay relationship," and he did not have children. "How should I treat my parents who are ashamed that I am gay?" he asked. "They seem to think that AIDS is a punishment. If they had truly accepted that there is nothing wrong with being gay, they wouldn't try to hide that I'm gay and have AIDS. I care about my parents, but I am angry at their insensitivity to me. Instead of feeling responsible to be a good son, I would like to focus on my own increasing needs because of AIDS and receive my parents' unconditional support."

"I'm trying to be as good a son as I can," Nate resolved. "Although I'm not happy that deep down they may always think being gay is wrong, I've tried to accept this."

Nate reasoned, "I want to contribute to my parents instead of giving them pain. I would like for them to see how my being gay and having AIDS can enrich their life, as it has enriched mine. Eventually, they are going to have to acknowledge that I am gay and have AIDS."

Commentary

The stories of Roger and Sally illustrate ethical problems involving HIV transmission from men to women to children. Roger questioned whether to have a baby by making a woman pregnant. To resolve his conflict, Roger said, "Ethically, that's not where I am today." Sally's conflict concerned whether to raise her newborn daughter who might be HIV-infected or let someone adopt the baby. She did not mention the baby's father. Describing her resolution, Sally said, "Right now, I'm planning her adoption. It's more important to do what's best for her than me."

Chapter 13 contains stories of women whose male sexual partners with AIDS were not as sexually responsible as Roger said that he was. Most women become HIV-infected by engaging in sex with men, after which they may pass the virus to their fetuses (CDC, 1992a).

As more women and children develop AIDS, associated ethical problems are attracting increasing public attention. Unfortunately, literature has focused on women and has overlooked men's responsibility for sexual behavior, pregnancy, and child rearing. Several ethical problems arise in the stories of Roger and Sally. Do HIV-infected persons have a right to produce children? If so, when one or more members of a couple are HIV-infected, should the couple be provided with infertility treatment (Smith et al., 1991)? Does society have the right or even obligation to intervene, coercively if necessary, to protect the unborn child (Gwin, 1991)?

In the United States, a growing trend is to use the law against parents who endanger their children. Prosecutors have charged some women with child abuse and neglect for abusing substances during pregnancy or at birth. Increasingly, judges have been willing to apply child abuse and neglect statutes in situations where a woman's behavior during pregnancy has resulted in physical or mental impairment of a child. Prosecution of women for maternal transmission of HIV disease to their babies might be the next step to protect children (Murphy, 1992).

In all probability, use of the law to punish women who bear HIV-infected children would be unjust and ineffective because it discriminates against women and does not take into account men's responsibility. Prosecutors would have difficulty establishing a woman's intentions regarding pregnancy and birth and the kinds of neglect or motive associated with legal culpability, especially since not all pregnancies end with an HIV-infected child. By using the law, prosecutors may not deter women with HIV disease from having children because pregnancy comes for many reasons beyond the reach of statutes and court judgments (Murphy, 1992).

Most ethicists have argued for other strategies than legal means to prevent HIV transmission from mothers to babies. One strategy is to stop viewing the maternal-fetal relationship as primarily adversarial in nature and see it as an interactive unit, where the needs of one help to define the needs of both. Balancing the needs of the mother and fetus is more likely to be helpful than punishing the mother (Faden et al., 1991; King, 1991; Mattingly, 1992; Steinbock, 1992).

A second strategy is to assure access to birth control and family planning. This intervention must be used with sensitivity and knowledge. Attempts to dissuade poor, low status, women of color from reproducing may be perceived as genocide (Almond & Ulanowsky, 1990; Bell, 1989; Hutchison & Kurth, 1991). Third, women could be routinely offered an HIV test before becoming pregnant, at an early stage of pregnancy, and after the baby's birth (Almond & Ulanowsky, 1990; Barbacci, Repke, & Chaisson, 1991). Then HIV-infected women would be able to obtain appropriate health care. Testing would permit women to assess possible outcomes of childbearing, even if such testing cannot predict individual outcomes exactly (Boyd, 1990; Heagarty & Abrams, 1992; Murphy, 1990; Powers, 1990; Walters, 1991).

A fourth strategy is to improve diagnosis of HIV-infected women. Often, HIV disease is not identified in women because health care personnel are reluctant to consider that a specific woman might be infected. Literature and research on HIV infection in women are sparse (Nokes, 1992).

Fifth, counseling could be used to reduce the likelihood of transmitting HIV disease from mothers to their babies. Counselors need to be knowledgeable about their clients' ethnic and socioeconomic background. They need skill to assist women and men to understand what reproduction means to them. Unfortunately, little research has been done on reproductive decision making among HIV-infected persons and those who are at risk for HIV disease (Hutchison & Kurth, 1991).

Finally, education is an intervention for preventing HIV transmission from mothers to their babies. Both women and men could be taught responsibility regarding sexuality, parenthood, and use of substances (Bayer, 1990). To be effective, educational offerings need to address the specific needs of the learners. Educators need to use language that learners understand and emphasize hope rather than fear (Williams, 1991).

The stories of Sally, Patsy, Conrad, Alice, and Belita illustrate ethical problems about minor children whose parents or grandparents have HIV disease. Questions arise regarding the emotional toll that parents' substance abuse, violence, criminal behavior, chronic illness, and death take on children. Who should care for children when their parents cannot? What kind of care should they be given? How should this care be financed?

These PWAs said that they did not want the state to remove their children or grandchildren from the home. As Belita put it, "Keep my family together would make my health better and my grandchildren happy." To keep the state from taking over care of her daughter, Sally was arranging her adoption. Alice said, "I got a lawyer through AIDS Foundation to write on paper that my half-sister would take my kids when I'm ready to die."

Patsy, Alice, Jane, and Wes described the conflict that parents can experience in explaining their diagnosis of AIDS to children. Alice asked, "How do you tell, 'Kids, I'm dying but I don't know when'?" Patsy said, "There's no good way to tell them without making them feel bad."

The other participants talked about the right way to balance their own needs and the needs of their partners, family, and friends. To resolve their conflict, they accounted for the needs of each person. "Part of the purpose of life is to make life better," said Helene, "and we make each other's lives better." Nate explained, "I want to contribute to my parents instead of giving them pain. I would like for them to see how my being gay and having AIDS can enrich their life, as it has enriched mine."

The participants' stories highlight difficulties that society has in providing social support for persons with HIV disease who are in nontraditional relationships. Because of AIDS, the gap between their needs and official designations of family has become apparent (Levine, 1990a). Often, traditional sources of social support are weak or nonexistent for them, and other sources are needed (Raveis & Siegel, 1991). A better approach than using legal means to punish HIV-infected persons would be to assist them to make responsible choices and develop supportive, long-lasting relationships.

Not only do persons who are HIV-infected need social support, but so do their loved ones. As indicated by Wes and Helene and documented in the literature, they may feel like the disease is controlling them instead of them managing the disease. They may be uncertain about how to live with loss and dying, changes in the relationship, dealing with other people, and preventing HIV transmission (Brown & Powell-Cope, 1991).

In summary, even though AIDS posed a serious threat, the participants expressed the desire for healthy, strong relationships. Todd spoke for several participants when he described what he was doing to enhance his connectedness with those whom they loved. "I am a good friend and supportive person," he said. "I have learned to like myself, and I'm one of my best friends. I love my family and friends dearly and pray that they will come to the same understanding that I have been blessed with. Being honest gives a wonderful feeling."

12

Ethical Problems Involving Service

AIDS activism grew out of the gay-rights movement. Early in the epidemic, most deaths from AIDS in the United States occurred among men who had sex with other men. By 1987, more than 20,000 Americans, about three fourths of them gay, had died of AIDS. Early hopes were dashed that the epidemic would be short-lived. The entire gay community was at risk. After HIV testing became available, tens of thousands of gay men were diagnosed as being HIV-positive. This evidence of their impending mortality imbued them with a passion to advocate on behalf of persons with HIV disease. They were outraged that the government and the health care system were not doing more about AIDS (Shilts, 1987).

Since then, AIDS activists have provided a service for HIV-infected persons and society by adding a new dimension to what was previously a polite dialogue among clinicians, researchers, policy makers, and advocates for health care clients. Actions of AIDS activists have varied from public demonstrations to detailed position papers and painstaking negotiation. The urgency and energy of AIDS activists have translated into expedited drug approvals, lower prices for medications, and increased funding for AIDS research and care (Campbell, 1991; Wachter, 1992).

Advocates for persons with other diseases have taken notice of AIDS activists. The rise in activism for breast cancer and Alzheimer's disease has resulted, in part, from success of the AIDS lobby. This activism is making fundamental changes in the health care system. No longer are some clients willing to be "patients," for they want to work in partnership with health care personnel (Brock, 1991; R. Levine, 1991; Wachter, 1992). Some of the participants engaged in AIDS activism by giving presentations, appearing on radio and television, publishing their stories, and producing videos and films. Five PWAs (one woman and four men) described ethical problems involving service: "Should I help other people or focus on myself?" "How should I balance being an AIDS activist and a PWA?"

"Should I Help Other People or Focus on Myself?"

MEG

Because Meg, a PWA, was concerned about confidentiality, I interviewed her in a basement room of an agency. She described conflict about whether to help other people or focus on herself.

"When I was first diagnosed with HIV," Meg said, "I wondered how this could be happening to me. I felt that I was the only one with HIV, that no one understood. I had to deal with people's lack of education about HIV. There are still myths. I wonder if going public about HIV could ruin stuff for me."

"I have decided to try to help other people with AIDS," Meg said about her resolution. "I've done videos, talks, a lot of outreach and education." She reasoned, "It's more important for me to educate people than to hide. Other people are going through the same thing as me and are afraid. The only thing I can do for myself and others is to educate them about AIDS. More people need to get involved. If they see other people doing AIDS education, maybe they will, too. Helping other people helps me feel better about myself. People helped me when I was first diagnosed, and I'm giving back what I received."

BRYAN

Bryan's ethical problem was similar to Meg's, except that he had AIDS and hemophilia. "Should I help other hemophilia(c)s who are infected with HIV even though I went through hell with the disease all by myself, except for my wife?" he asked. "No one told me that if you become short of breath, you're getting pneumonia. I didn't know why I would get a rash, and it would go away a day later. Until recently, I would never talk about having AIDS. I was so scared, I wouldn't even go to the doctor."

Bryan described his resolution to his conflict. "My first exposure to helping was with my friend," he said. "I assisted him to accept the disease and himself. I should find one guy with hemophilia and have him tested so he doesn't infect somebody else like his wife. I've been invited to speak to classes. At first, I was afraid to tell my mother that I have AIDS, but now I'm getting to the point where I think I can. I could start a support group for hemophilia(c)s with AIDS."

"I feel a calling to help other hemophilia(c)s who are infected with HIV," reasoned Bryan. "I don't want them to go through the pain and denial that I went through. Formerly, I didn't care about people. I wasn't going to do anything about stopping the spread of AIDS. But now that I have AIDS, I don't want anybody else to get it. Everybody has a right to life. I want to help even one person say, 'I'll put on a condom.' If I help someone not contract AIDS or be afraid of AIDS, I've done something good. I would rather help other people than help myself. I've grown since getting AIDS."

SCOTT

Scott, a PWA who was recovering from an opportunistic infection, said, "My presentation about AIDS tends to make a conference a success. Celebrity status comes because people are drawn to a story of someone infected versus an educator's point of view. But egos have gotten in the way. AIDS educators have been doing the work on a regular basis. When I come on the scene, and I am infected, what I say is more dynamic than what they say, and I get more attention. They feel that this threatens their program, their celebrity status. It takes away from them having the podium. When it gets back to me, I've been made to feel, 'Who are you?' That's painful. I'm trying to do good, and they are criticizing me. When they treat me like that, why not say, 'To hell with this work. Why should I continue?' "

"When I feel down," Scott said about his resolution, "I look at the letters from students. My presentations have made a difference in their sexual practices and concerns. Reading these letters gives me an incentive, the drive to continue with what I'm doing. They lift me right back up because they say, 'Keep up the good work. We need more people like you.' "

Explaining his rationale for his resolution, Scott said, "The students write that they've had education by health educators, seen things on television and in newspapers, and they've read brochures. But none of those made a difference until they saw me. That's the highest high that someone can get from doing this work. It means I have succeeded if even one person is changing. What I say takes away the fear that they had in the pit of their stomach in relating to someone with AIDS. That encouragement gives me the motivation to keep working with these AIDS educators and dealing with the politics of AIDS."

"How Should I Balance Being an AIDS Activist and a Person With AIDS?"

BURT

Burt, a PWA, was a nurse, although he did not work full time because of health problems. "As a nurse, should I choose to be right and stand up for what I believe or reduce stress in my life so that I stay healthy?" he asked. "Should I help the disenfranchised and AIDS service organizations or work the system to get my needs met? A person in my support group complains of eye trouble, and the physician says to get new glasses, when it is AIDS-related. I take on many tackles like this. My health can be jeopardized if the fight consumes me, and the stress is so great that I lose sleep or I'm not eating right."

Burt described his resolution to his conflict. "I work hard at being a good caregiver and taking care of myself," he said. "I take time outs when I become too involved, and I've learned to guard my involvement in projects because I've burned out. I resolve situations on a case-by-case basis. I did AIDS Hospice and AIDS education because nobody was doing them. But when other people did them, I could stop. I've developed policy."

"Ever since becoming a nurse," Burt said, explaining his rationale, "I've wanted to help other people. There's a call to being a nurse. I'm invested in enhancing quality of life for all people including myself. A sense of integrity comes, provided I take care of myself. Then the balance is healthy. Helping other people is empowering. It enhances the quality of my life by giving me purpose, meaning, satisfaction. Otherwise, why stay alive? We have gross ethical inequities in the system and I'm going to do what I can to make things better because that's what I do. It helps me pay the bills."

"There is a lack of collaboration between service organizations and the PWA population," Burt continued. "These organizations have hundreds of thousands of dollars in grants to do a study that has been done or is proven not to work, and yet they don't have money for our needs. I believe in collaboration. Reallocating things and having one case manager for each client is more equitable, and each client isn't going to five organizations. Only some of our potential is actualized because of politics, turf fighting, and misinterpretation of need."

LUKE

While answering phone calls, Luke questioned how to balance being an AIDS activist and a PWA. "I feel conflict between my roles as a long-term survivor with AIDS and a PWA advocate," he began. "I need to take care of myself, but I'm also the director of an AIDS agency, a group facilitator, a speaker, and a leader in a national organization. Do I call a sick client every day? Doing so for all of my clients would be a full-time occupation."

"Because I advocate for people with their doctors," Luke continued, "I am having trouble replacing my doctor who moved away. It's hard to find a doctor who will treat me as a person with AIDS, not the director of an agency. Where can I get emotional support for myself? People who are on the front line giving support to PWAs, like myself, are not getting the support they need because they can't get involved in a particular organization. Sometimes I feel conflict with other AIDS activists, or I run myself ragged supporting the rights of other people with AIDS, but I don't get their support."

"I feel conflict because confidentiality is getting out of hand," said Luke. "Nurses, doctors, and social workers cannot get the support they need, and they are getting burned out. I feel conflict between people who are dealing with holistic, spiritual, well-being approaches and people who are in the mode of taking orders from doctors. I think both approaches go hand-in-hand. Doctors don't agree about what terms to use, and there is confusion about medications and when to intervene. I feel conflict because people who are newly diagnosed don't try to help their brothers and sisters with AIDS."

"I feel conflict about how to deal with the many groups involved with AIDS," Luke went on, "each of which thinks that its agenda is most important. Instead of working as a family unit, everyone is fighting for rights, housing, medical treatment for their group. Women, children, and people of color with AIDS have not had proper treatment. By being divided into competing groups, we're throwing more oppression onto the disease."

"The most damaging thing has been the politics of AIDS," Luke said, "more than having AIDS. Is it crazy to do what I'm doing, having AIDS myself, and being an unpaid volunteer? Why do it when people are taking advantage of the system? Why not take care of myself? Some people with AIDS have written books, done videos, have made money off of people with AIDS. Should I?"

Luke described his resolution to his conflict. "My health is changing," he said, "and I'm looking for new people to come in and take responsibility. I am considering doing political advocacy less on a local level and more on a national level."

"I'm learning to tell myself that conflict with other people isn't my problem," he said. "Instead of looking on the negative aspect of stress, I've learned how to use it in a positive way. I set limits for myself. People have to understand I am the director of a business. Since I can't be there for everyone, part of their empowerment is to ask to see me instead of expecting me. When I counsel people who complain about the system, I tell them how lucky they are. If they had other diseases, they wouldn't have housing, meals, buddy programs. If they want better services, they should get involved."

"You can't be liked by all people," Luke reasoned. "Since all of us make mistakes, we might as well accept each other. There are many choices, but no right way to deal with AIDS. The only thing is open your heart and give as much compassion as you can. People are seeking help because of the lack of support that they're getting in their families. I believe in unconditional love, loving yourself fully, accepting who you are."

"It's important to resolve conflict and not let it bottle up," Luke continued. "Otherwise, it's going to put more stress on you. Being an AIDS activist is a lot of stress, but it's also new challenges each day and helps me to live well with AIDS. The venting helps me let go of stress. I'm keeping active. I'm not using the system. I'm leaving a mark on something. I've accepted the death process as part of the living process. The quality of life we have until we die is most important. I've survived so long with AIDS because of my activism."

Commentary

As the PWAs' stories illustrate, AIDS activists may experience four kinds of conflicts: conflicts among PWAs, conflicts between PWAs and providers of services, conflicts between AIDS activists and society, and conflicts within society. In spite of good intentions, AIDS activists may add to and be caught in the middle of these tensions. If they are HIV-infected themselves, their health may suffer from "the politics of AIDS."

Conflicts among PWAs may arise because of increasing diversity in the AIDS community. No longer do PWAs consist primarily of Caucasian men who have sex with men, but they are also heterosexuals, injecting drug users, and people of color. "I feel conflict about how to deal with the many groups involved with AIDS," Luke explained, "each of which thinks that its agenda is most important. By being divided into different competing groups, we're throwing more oppression onto the disease."

To effectively resolve conflicts among PWAs, AIDS activists must confront poverty, racism, sexism, homophobia, violence, substance abuse, teenage pregnancy, and poor access to health care. Strategies that were effective among Caucasian gay men may not be appropriate for other groups. Different strategies may be needed that take into account the cultures, languages, and institutions of AIDS-impacted individuals (Wachter, 1992).

Second, AIDS activists may experience conflicts between PWAs and providers of services. Suggesting how to resolve these conflicts, Burt said, "I believe in collaboration. Reallocating things and having one case manager for each client is more equitable, and each client isn't going to five organizations."

Third, AIDS activists may experience conflicts between themselves and society. The AIDS lobby has not been universally praised. AIDS activists have been criticized for using militant tactics and for alienating their natural allies, such as clinicians and scientists. Critics contend that AIDS activists inadequately embrace the viewpoints of diverse groups at risk for HIV disease (Campbell, 1991; Wachter, 1992).

Some critics have argued that because of AIDS activists, HIV disease is given exceptional treatment in public policy as far as testing, screening, reporting, notifying partners, and prosecuting persons whose behavior threatens to transmit the virus. Public sentiment seems to be growing that HIV disease gets more than its fair share of resources (Bayer, 1991). Luke himself called PWAs "lucky," saying, "If they had other diseases, they wouldn't have housing, meals, buddy programs."

AIDS activists will need to deal directly with these criticisms to counteract a backlash against AIDS. Certainly, the participants' stories illustrate that HIV disease is a disaster. The virus has turned intimate forms of human contact into a means for transmitting a lethal disease. HIV infection will not go away by wishing that people would refrain from risky behavior. The number of persons being diagnosed with the disease continues to rise, and more and scarcer resources have to be directed to caring for them (Cooper & Weiss, 1989; Murphy, 1991b).

Rather than talk about special treatment for HIV-infected individuals, advocates for persons with Alzheimer's disease, cancer, heart disease, and other conditions could join AIDS activists and form a powerful coalition of consumers. These groups have in common a number of issues, such as discrimination and health care access (Wachter, 1992). If these groups do not collaborate, health care policy could become increasingly fractious and even hazardous. Powerful groups could succeed in garnering larger slices of the resource pie, whereas equally deserving groups could be left with smaller slices because they do not have activists to lobby on their behalf (Wachter, 1992).

Finally, AIDS activists may experience conflicts within society, a major source of contention being AIDS education. Nearly everyone agrees that people should be told about HIV disease. However, consensus does not exist about the content of AIDS education, how early to begin it, to which groups it should be directed, who should teach it, and how long it should continue. Some people argue for AIDS education that is frank and sexually explicit, such as teaching learners how to make sexual activity and drug use safer. Critics contend that such approaches legitimate or give approval to activities that are thought to be morally (and at times, legally) wrong (Bell, 1991).

Because education seems to be the best hope at this time for dealing with HIV disease (Strauss, Corless, Luckey, van der Horst, & Dennis, 1992), AIDS activists will need to work with society to resolve unanswered questions about AIDS education. With government funding, research can continue to be conducted about what type of AIDS education is most effective (Cooper & Weiss, 1989). Including content about ethics in AIDS education will help learners to become knowledgeable about ethical problems involving AIDS, and they may be better able to resolve them. Discussions of codependency will highlight risks of engaging in unprotected sex as a result of an addictive relationship when HIV infection is involved (St. Onge, 1992).

Research suggests that effective AIDS education helps learners to understand how words and images attach negative messages to the disease (Watney, 1987). Teachers convey information in an understandable, scientifically accurate manner that fosters individual responsibility (Cooper & Weiss, 1989). Programs are provided for adolescents, older persons, people of color, women, persons with little education, and men having unprotected sex with men or women, regardless of their sexual identity (Fielstein, Fielstein, & Hazelwood, 1992; McCaig, Hardy, & Winn, 1991). These programs take into account social and cultural influences affecting sexual behavior and identity (Doll et al., 1992). Offering HIV testing and counseling as part of AIDS education may facilitate behavior change (Boekeloo et al., 1991; Silverman, Perakyla, & Bor, 1992; Wenger, Linn, Epstein, & Shapiro, 1991; Zenilman, Erickson, Fox, Reichart, & Hook, 1992).

Facing these conflicts, many AIDS activists have jeopardized their own health. Not only do activists with HIV disease have to deal with the disease process, but they also may experience burnout because of the "politics of AIDS." Perhaps the greatest challenge to activism comes from burnout and the merciless nature of HIV disease. Many HIV-infected activists have been lost to the movement through burnout, illness, and death (Wachter, 1992).

Like activists with HIV disease, non-HIV-infected activists and care providers in the AIDS community can become burned out (Eakes, 1990). "I feel conflict because confidentiality is getting out of hand," said Luke. "Nurses, doctors, and social workers cannot get the support that they need, and they are getting burned out."

Burnout is a combination of emotional exhaustion, depersonalization, and reduced personal accomplishment, which may be a consequence of the chronic stressors of daily life (Driedger & Cox, 1991). When one feels unable to give any more psychologically, emotional exhaustion occurs. Depersonalization results from cynical and negative attitudes that affect one's feelings regarding clients. Reduced personal accomplishment arises from the tendency to evaluate oneself negatively, especially in regard to clients (Driedger & Cox, 1991).

Research suggests that social support can provide a coping mechanism for avoiding and recovering from burnout. Social support tends to insulate people from the effects of job stress. For some people in the field of HIV disease, participating in a support group has decreased their symptoms of burnout (Driedger & Cox, 1991; Kendall, 1992; Knox & Gaies, 1992; Stein et al., 1991; Tannebaum & Butler, 1992).

Another way to reduce burnout is through conflict management (Driedger & Cox, 1991; Tannebaum & Butler, 1992). Scott explained that when he felt stress, he read what students at his presentations wrote to him. Luke said, "Instead of looking on the negative aspect of stress, I've learned how to use it in a positive way."

AIDS activists have worked hard to resolve conflicts. They have stimulated the government to address some needs of AIDS-impacted persons, monitored government shortcomings, attempted to fill in the gap for what government cannot or will not do (Kobasa, 1990), and encouraged HIV-infected persons to no longer see themselves as "patients" but work collaboratively with providers of services. Explaining what he told PWAs who complained about the "system," Luke said, "If they want better services, they should get involved."

Moreover, another form of AIDS activism has appeared. AIDS has spawned many creative works in the arts and mass media that bring society into contact with the emotional impact of the disease (Goldstein, 1990). As shared, communal experiences, these works give concrete, individual form to ethical problems that otherwise could be elusively abstract (Cady & Hunter, 1989; Murphy & Poirier, 1993).

In summary, despite many difficulties involving activism, the PWAs said that speaking out publicly was preferable to remaining silent, as long as they took into account their health. As Burt put it, "Helping other people enhances the quality of my life by giving me purpose, meaning, satisfaction." Luke said, "I've survived so long with AIDS because of my activism."

13

Ethical Problems Involving Sexuality

The most common ways to transmit HIV disease are through vaginal and anal sexual intercourse. Mucosal tissues of the vagina and rectum are rich in superficial blood vessels. If these tissues have small tears, white blood cells harboring the virus that come into contact with the tissues can enter the host's blood stream (Green, 1987).

To reduce the possibility of HIV transmission, public health officials have advised people to take responsibility for their sexual behavior. They have suggested that HIV-infected persons abstain from sexual intercourse or engage in sex with fully informed adults who use precautions. For persons without HIV disease, public health officials have recommended abstinence or monogamous sex with a non-HIV-infected partner. If these options are not likely, non-HIV-infected individuals should use protection when engaging in sex, have few sexual partners, and talk openly with their sexual partners about AIDS (CDC, 1992b; Cline, Johnson, & Freeman, 1992).

Although the fear of AIDS has prompted some individuals to alter their sexual behavior, other people have not seemed to change, even after being told about modes of HIV transmission. Research indicates that teenagers may be engaging in unsafe sex at nearly the same rate as before AIDS was first identified (Brooks-Gunn & Furstenberg, 1990; CDC, 1992b). Women may want to use protection, but they

may feel they have little personal power to demand that men use
condoms (Bell, 1989). The self-esteem of some men who have sex
with men may be so low because of society's homophobia that they
take part in abusive sex. Persons who are under the influence of
alcohol and drugs may not be able to make responsible choices about
their sexual activities (Crimp, 1988; Eliason & Randall, 1991).

All of the participants seemed knowledgeable about modes of
HIV transmission. Figure 13.1 describes their sex practices. Fourteen
PWAs (4 women and 10 men) and three significant persons specifically described ethical problems involving sexuality: "Should I engage in protected sex or unprotected sex?" "Should I be concerned
about my partner's sexuality or focus on my own sexual needs?"
"Should I accept or reject that I am gay?" "Should I be sexual as a
gay man even though I may infect someone with HIV?" "Should
I be sexual as a heterosexual person even though I may infect
someone with HIV?"

"Should I Engage in Protected Sex or Unprotected Sex?"

ROXANNE

Roxanne, who became HIV-infected from "heterosexual sex,"
described conflict about whether she should engage in protected
or unprotected sex. "Should I care about transmitting HIV to
someone else?" she asked. "A lot of people think somebody gave
them AIDS, and they're going to give it to everybody. They fuck
everybody and don't give a fart. They are getting venereal diseases,
and it's killing them faster. I don't want that to happen to me."

Describing her resolution to her conflict, Roxanne said, "I use
condoms and avoid becoming infected by someone else." She
rationalized, "I can't afford to catch anything from anybody or be
infected with the virus again because that breaks my system down
twice as fast. I don't want to be the cause of somebody dying
because life is precious." After blowing her nose, she said, "My
tears are because people don't take life seriously."

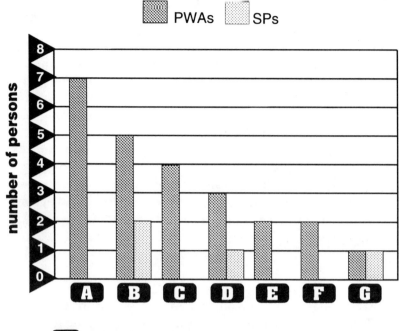

A   Celibate Past 6 Months
B   Always Uses Condoms with Jelly
C   Always Uses Condoms
D   Sometimes Uses Condoms
E   Does Not Exchange Body Fluids
F   Engages in Lesbian Sex
G   Does Not Use Any Protection

Figure 13.1. Self-Reported Descriptions of 25 Persons With AIDS (PWAs) and 5 Significant Persons (SPs) About Their Sex Practices

ANDY

Andy became HIV-infected from blood products to treat his hemophilia. "Should I use condoms with women that I date?" he asked. "Should I tell them about HIV? I'm afraid to. They might reject me. Should I use condoms with my present girlfriend? She found out about me being infected and got bent out of shape."

"When I was dating other women," Andy said of his resolution, "I told them about HIV. The ones that wanted a condom, didn't make a difference to me. I felt that we can do this to keep you safe. With my present girlfriend, sometimes we use condoms, and sometimes we don't, the emotion at the moment."

Andy reasoned, "If I didn't have HIV, I wouldn't want nobody giving it to me. You might be taking a life, and that's wrong. I am a good person and don't want to hurt nobody. Before sexual encounters, it's best to let women know what they're up against so they can decide if it matters. I wish I could have made a decision about getting HIV."

SHARI

Shari, a significant person and Andy's girlfriend, described conflict about whether to use protection when engaging sex. "For the first 6 months we were together," she said, "I didn't know he's infected, and we didn't use condoms. I found out by overhearing him on the phone, and I cried. In my mind, he was saying he didn't care if he got me infected. We talked, but he refuses to use condoms, and I'm afraid I will become infected. I don't want to get AIDS because I have children. One is disabled. He's more comfortable without condoms. All men are like that."

"If it's only me and him," Shari continued, "I'm not afraid of AIDS. I found him with another female. He said it was his friend's girlfriend. I hope he don't be like all men and most females and want to share himself with someone else. I'm respecting him as a human being, not a diseased person, and he can respect me as a female. I have needs, being in the relationship one-on-one."

Shari described her resolution. "We don't use condoms," she said. "I go to the doctor to make sure I haven't gotten HIV. He's not planning to be with a girl no more than a night or couple of days, but I take it one step at a time."

Explaining her rationale for her resolution, Shari said, "Men or females with HIV should tell their partner in an adult way. AIDS shouldn't be spread to anyone else. Since I'm risking my life by having sex with him without condoms, I want him to be faithful. If I wanted to use condoms, he'd be willing, but I don't want nothing to be uncomfortable for him. I think more of him than myself. It doesn't bother me that we don't use condoms, because I go to the doctor regularly. If you're going to get AIDS, you're going to get AIDS. We all got to go some day."

"Should I Be Concerned About My Partner's Sexuality or Focus on My Own Sexual Needs?"

DIANA

When Diana was in jail, she tested positive for HIV disease. She had not engaged in sex with her boyfriend, who injected drugs, for 2½ months because "I don't feel good enough," and she questioned whether to be concerned about his sexuality or focus on her own.

"I'm worried about my boyfriend passing HIV to somebody," Diana said. "He gave HIV to me, I wasn't messing around. AIDS is deadly, and I wouldn't want it to happen to someone else."

Diana said about her resolution, "I told him, 'I'm too sick to have sex with you, and if you go elsewhere, you'd better use a rubber, and make sure it's safe for the other person.' He promised he'd keep rubbers on him. I ask him, 'Have you had sex with anybody?' I told him, 'Rubbers not safe, they break.' "

"My boyfriend is a man," Diana reasoned, "and I can't expect him not to have sex because I don't have sex. I'm too scared to have sex with anyone but my boyfriend because I don't want to pass HIV on. That would be too much to keep having sex and passing HIV on."

MARGO

"I don't know how I got it," Margo said about HIV disease. "My husband doesn't know he got it, either." She described conflict similar to Diana's conflict.

"My husband has a high sex drive," Margo said. "He got to have sex, if it's four times a day, 7 days a week. When a man is not satisfied, he's going to go somewhere else and get it. Both of us having AIDS has slowed him down, but I'm worried that he could spread the illness to someone else."

"I told him, 'Sex is there whenever you want it,' " Margo said, describing her resolution. "You have to be cautious to avoid HIV to be spread more.' My sexual needs is, if I get it, fine. If I don't, it don't bother me. My husband is generous. He has never said, 'You can't have any,' or make an excuse. What we're doing about sex seems to be working. We have sex, but we use condoms. We don't have sex as much as we used to. It's monogamous, so we don't pass it on or bring something back."

"I rather him stay here and get sex," Margo rationalized. "That help me with my own sexual needs. A wife is for her husband alone. A husband is for a wife alone. It's not to be shared. It's breaking a commitment. I am serious about my marriage vows and my relationship with my husband."

CHRIS

Chris, a significant person, explained that his wife had become HIV-infected from a blood transfusion during surgery, which took place before blood was tested for HIV disease. He described conflict about whether to be concerned about his wife's sexuality or concentrate on his own sexual needs.

"I want to be sexually satisfied," Chris began, "but HIV makes me scared of sex with my wife, and protection limits my sexual satisfaction. I am concerned that I will lose an erection because of the condom. Sometimes I am tired or stressed. That's when the darn condom is a headache and helps to make me a failure, which is rare. Then she feels bad for me. Do I look elsewhere for sexual

satisfaction? I am pulled between my love for her and desire to remain monogamous and my wish to be sexually fulfilled."
"My heart goes out to her, and her heart goes out to me," Chris said about his resolution. "We made a game of finding the best condom. Some were sloppy, messy, smelly. We found a thin, sensitive one that is more satisfactory. Now we always use condoms and jelly, and we've never broken one yet. She tries to compensate for their limitations. We are careful about washing. Our living is close to normal. We avoid having sex when we are overly tired or stressed. HIV hasn't diminished our sex life."
Chris explained his rationale, saying, "While condoms are not as satisfying as regular intercourse, they're better than nothing. Sex is only one part of the relationship. The right thing to do is be monogamous and live in harmony with our values. Having an affair or picking up a prostitute would be shallow. Why us? There isn't an answer. It's happenstance. You take the good with the bad, and accept what you can't change. Struggling with adversity is part of growing."

"Should I Accept or Reject That I Am Gay?"

THEO

When I asked Theo, a PWA, how he became HIV-infected, he said, "Ninety-nine percent chance gay sex and one percent needles." He explained that he and his life partner, who was not HIV-infected, used protection during sex. Eager to talk, he said, "I don't have anything to fear from people knowing." As we sat in his kitchen, he questioned whether to accept being gay.
"I lived most of my life feeling bad about being different," said Theo. "Like other gay boys and lesbian girls, I grew up in a heterosexual environment that is biased against homosexuality. We develop a strong gay or lesbian sexual identity in spite of rejection. I tried to change so people would love me, but I couldn't change being gay. Should I be honest about who I am?"

Theo described his resolution. "When I realized there was a name—gay—for what I was, that I could be proud of, I liked myself better," he said. "Hating myself didn't get me anywhere. I decided to love myself and be honest. Now I embrace my differences. I told my family that I was gay, and they didn't reject me. I am open with other people about being gay."

"I can't be the person everybody wants me to be," rationalized Theo. "I have to be me. Differences aren't bad, they are wonderful. Being gay doesn't make me a bad person. Most people like me even though they know I am gay. If it's too big of an issue for them, they make their choice."

LEWIS

Lewis become HIV-infected from "gay sex." He had not had sex for "1 year" but would engage in "safe sex." Unlike Theo, he was concerned about confidentiality, and we met secretly.

"The conflict is that I've been gay all my life," Lewis said. "But if I wasn't gay, would I have gotten AIDS? Before I became educated, I morally thought that AIDS was punishment from God. I fight that issue. People have said to me, 'You chose this life-style, and AIDS is what you have to live with.' Society has put stigma on gay people."

"When the voice inside says, 'If you hadn't been gay, you wouldn't have AIDS,' I answer with hope, strength, God," Lewis said about his resolution. "I say, 'I didn't choose to be gay. This is who I am.' I fight harder to stay alive and be healthy. I go with the flow and deal with it the best I know how."

Explaining his rationale, Lewis said, "People feel that if you weren't gay, AIDS wouldn't have happened. And that's sad. It makes a difference to me that AIDS can happen to anyone, and I'm not alone with AIDS. I'm a spiritual person. I was raised in church. God is an important part of my life, which gives me strength and hope. God knows all, and I don't think that AIDS is God's fault. AIDS isn't a punishment."

"Should I Be Sexual as a Gay Man Even Though I May Infect Someone With HIV?"

JACOB

Jacob, who became HIV-infected from "gay sex," described conflict about whether he should be sexual as a gay man. "As an Afro-American man growing up," he began, "it's important to experiment with sex. In the homosexual life-style, at least in the past, we tend to have more than one partner, which is like sleeping with a community of people. A lot of us are careless with sex. We say, 'They didn't look out for me, so why should I look out for them?' Should I be sexually involved with someone else and take the chance of infecting that person?"

"I want to be more aware, responsible, cautious about sex," Jacob resolved. "Unfortunately, I haven't been involved with someone because of AIDS. I like to keep my relationships to a minimum. To be fair, I want to be involved with someone who's also infected so I don't infect anyone else. An infected person will know what AIDS is like."

"I care about whether people get HIV because someone didn't care about me," Jacob reasoned. "If I had considered myself, I wouldn't have AIDS. It's important to care about other people and yourself. If you're a sexually responsible person, you protect yourself and the other person. By taking a few minutes, you won't get AIDS. You can be responsible regardless of your age or color."

MARTIN

When I asked Martin, a PWA, how he became HIV-infected, he replied, "Gay sex." He began, "At a young age, I realized I was attracted to men or boys but fought it and pursued heterosexual relationships. After graduating from high school, I resolved to be true to my sexuality. When diagnosed with HIV, I had a death wish and did not offer people the choice for life if I had sex with them in an unsafe manner. I felt guilty that some people I'd had sexual relationships with died. When I didn't die, too, I thought I was a fluke. I needed affection and intimacy and didn't know how to get them. My feelings were too much."

"I learned the ethics of Alcoholics Anonymous," Martin said about his resolution, "and found I had been dishonest with potential sex partners. I redefined my boundaries as they relate to intimacy, and now I engage in safe sex. I'm true to my sexuality and have a gay lover."

Explaining his rationale for his resolution, Martin said, "Sexuality is who I am. A warm hug is as important as copulation. From my relationship with my lover, I'm learning that sexuality and sexual intercourse aren't the same. I don't have to be who everyone says a gay or sexual person is. I have to be myself, doing what feels good, safe, responsible."

ERIC

Eric, who had become HIV-infected from "needles or gay sex," asked, "How should I meet my sexual needs in a manner that isn't destructive to me or anyone else but promotes my spiritual growth? I associate naughty sex with fun, just like society that rates movies according to sexual content. How should I be sexual without a naughty element? Can I keep AIDS from taking away my sexuality? AIDS screwed up having sex because I must do things to prevent transmission, and I have to fight the desire to engage in unprotected sex. What should I recommend to people about disclosing their HIV status to potential sex partners? People who are honest about their HIV status may be rejected."

"I am a sexual person through nurturing, love, respect, and sharing," Eric described his resolution to his conflict. "Raunchiness, deception, control, and naughtiness are not part of me anymore. I am sexually active in my monogamous relationship. I won't endanger my partner if I don't engage in activities that transmit HIV. Protected sex becomes normal. I tell people to be honest with potential sex partners about their HIV status, and they are successful, with few exceptions."

Eric reasoned, "Being gay doesn't make me a bad person. Sex doesn't need a nasty element to be fun. Sex isn't bad, it's a wonderful gift. HIV-infected persons build relationships that are loving with noninfected persons, and people start relationships with HIV-infected persons. Even though society has marked us for death, these people see that we are persons, and they love us. They're having rich, full relationships."

BRUCE

Bruce became HIV-infected from "gay sex, good sex!" Although celibate for 4 years, he questioned whether to be sexual even though he could infect someone with HIV disease.

"When I was diagnosed," Bruce began, "I wanted to share HIV with everybody. 'Fuck the doctors.' I had unsafe, casual sex. As an Asian Pacific gay man, I didn't love myself and wanted to use sex to validate myself. Having sex was a cultural sharing with my sub, sub-culture, being Pacific Islander and gay. I don't do that now, but I wonder, should I have a sexual relationship with my friends? Should I be honest with my parents about my sexuality and AIDS? I'm the oldest son and heir to what my parents built. I don't want them to suffer."

"How should I deal with the unfairness of AIDS and its effect on my sexuality?" he asked. "Death is coming soon for me. I am at the peak of my career. I have a lot to give, smiles for people, lovely things to say to clerks who work in stores on days when they should be off. I want better. That's a lot to ask."

"After my lover died," Bruce said about his resolution, "I was hospitalized, and they told me I was going to die. I woke up, and my room was bathed in an eerie, orange glow. A Filipino woman was wiping night sweat from my body and saying, 'God loves you.' God was talking to me, and the simple message was, if God loves me, I can love myself enough to take care of myself and not engage in this emotional, spiritual, physical self-flagellation, and not endanger others. When I got out of the hospital, I went back and asked to speak to the Filipino nurse. There was no Filipino nurse on duty that night."

"I decided to stop engaging in casual, unprotected sex," said Bruce. "I become celibate and an AIDS activist. I had to get a grip on myself, accept responsibilities taught to me as a child. I said, 'Bubba, stop this bullshit. It's stupid. Doesn't help. Makes the situation worse. Do the best you can. See your doctor every month. Take the medications.' I talked to my mother, and put all my cards on the table."

Bruce reasoned, "Engaging in self-flagellation isn't the cure for AIDS because AIDS is still here. I don't want to make somebody sick. I am not a destroyer of life. I became celibate because no matter how many condoms you use, the virus can get through. Sometimes people use protection, sometimes not. My friends and I don't know who infected who, a sorrowful situation. Many of them have died, and I have grief issues about them."

"The gay community denies discrimination toward Asian Pacific Islanders," Bruce continued. "Rice queens, white men who are into Asian Pacific men, brought the virus into our culture. Generally, they are aggressive or top and easily pass the infection to the passive or bottom. The Centers for Disease Control say that only a few Asian Pacific Islanders are infected, so we don't get money to fight AIDS. But almost all of us are infected. Death certificates don't say AIDS. They say pneumonia or heart insufficiency. I became an activist because no Asian Pacific Islander was saying a word about AIDS. So I am going to make a difference if I can."

"Should I Be Sexual as a Heterosexual Person Even Though I May Infect Someone With HIV?"

MARILYN

Marilyn, who became HIV-infected from "heterosexual sex," described conflict about being sexual. "I long for a companion to love me, AIDS and all," she said. "You can enjoy sex, laugh. You a person. But do you want to tell that person about AIDS? That could be tough. I might never see him again. He may reject me if I insist on condoms. One man, I insisted on condoms. He said it didn't matter to him, he wasn't afraid of HIV. I said it did matter to me. So he didn't want to have sex with me."

"I'm young," Marilyn resolved, "but I'm refraining from sex now. I am looking for a long-term companion. If I find him, I will tell him about HIV and use protection when we have sex."

Explaining her rationale, Marilyn said, "You have to tell him about AIDS to give you peace inside. A person have a right to know. Keeping a secret is not telling who you are. It's like being pregnant with another man's baby, and you meet this guy, and you not showing. A relationship need to be based on honesty, not a lie. I would use protection because I don't want to destroy nobody, or I couldn't live with myself. Because of AIDS, I may have to live without a companion."

TONIO

Tonio became HIV-infected from a blood transfusion to treat his hemophilia before blood products were tested for HIV. "I take precautions to not infect my wife," he began, "but I'm concerned that they will not work. Sexual intercourse dropped after my diagnosis with HIV and even more with AIDS. I have a psychological blockage because there's a chance of transmission. Condoms are a pain because your brain has to be working so you don't get carried away, and it says, 'Should you be doing this?' "

Tonio described his resolution to his conflict. "We use protected sex," he said, "and wait until we want to have sex rather than force it. My physician said my blockage was probably psychological. Rationalization took over, and for awhile we were able to do it. Now it's infrequent again, but it's not true impotence any more. I don't perform like I did when we were first married. That falls off normally in a married couple."

"My psychological blockage may not be due entirely to AIDS," Tonio said, explaining his rationale, "because the males in my family were never over-sexed. Sex is important, and we don't want to give it up, but it isn't the most important part of our relationship. Having sex less often hasn't affected our relationship. If anything it's firmer than before AIDS."

RAYMOND

Raymond, too, became HIV-infected from a blood transfusion to treat his hemophilia. "I want to have sex with my wife," he said, "but I don't want to infect her, and this fear affects our marriage. We have cut back on sex from a couple of times a week to every couple of months. All the precautions spoil the spontaneity. She asks to have sex, but something in me says, 'You can't.' When I got AIDS, it got worse. I can't handle the pressure of sex. I should have sex whenever it comes up, but I don't do that. Since sex is hard, I wonder if it's worth it."

"It's crazy," he said about his resolution, "but we use two condoms and a spermicide gel. When I break down, I have sex with her, but not as often as we'd like. As I accept having AIDS, it's easier on our sexual relationship. She's accepted it. It's coming with time. We're working on it."

"Not infecting my wife, or anyone else, is most important," Raymond reasoned. "If I infected her, I couldn't live with myself. I'd go crazy. I care more about her than I do for myself at most times because of the love she's given me. Breaking down to have sex is the wrong way of looking at it. I won't have sex with someone else, though."

VANCE

Vance, who became HIV-infected from a blood transfusion to treat his hemophilia, said that he was unmarried but in a long-time relationship with his girlfriend. "What is the right way to meet my sexual needs?" he asked. "For a young male, sex is way up there on the list of priorities, especially after a couple of drinks. Should I have a sexual relationship with my girlfriend? Protected sex is still dangerous, and I don't want to infect her. Should I be monogamous with her, or have a primary relationship with her while having relationships with other women? I want to be honest with her, but I don't want her to know about my relationships with other women, or she might leave me. I want to keep my present girlfriend, yet I am attracted to other women."

"Before having sex with another woman, should I tell her that I have AIDS?" Vance asked. "I don't want to ruin my chances with her. Should I do what is ethically right or what brings me immediate physical gratification? How can I meet my sexual needs without hurting her? Is it right to pursue a sexual relationship knowing the risk that she is taking?"

"Usually, I use condoms when I have sex with my girlfriend, but they break or fall off," Vance about his resolution to his conflict. "I engaged in unprotected sex with my former girlfriend before and after I found out that I was HIV-positive. Since she hadn't become infected previously, I figured she wouldn't become infected by having sex a few more times. When my buddy and I met a couple of women, I opted for immediate physical gratification. I had sexual relations with one of them without exactly telling her the situation, but I was careful."

"Since the relationship with my present girlfriend is improving, I have less desire for sex with other women, and I don't feel as much conflict," Vance rationalized. "It's important to use protected sex. I should tell a woman that I have AIDS before having sex with her. It is unethical to have sex, even if it is protected sex, without telling her that I have AIDS. It's not fair to her because she doesn't know that she is potentially risking her life."

LISA

Lisa, a significant person and Vance's girlfriend, said that they did not consistently use condoms, and she questioned whether to be sexual with him even though she might become HIV-infected herself. Although she brought up the topic about sex, she seemed self-conscious to talk about it. She gave only a brief description before turning to another ethical problem.

"I love him and want a sexual relationship with him," explained Lisa, "but by having sex with him, I could get AIDS." Describing her resolution, she said, "I have a sexual relationship with him, and usually we use condoms." She reasoned, "I'm fine having a sexual relationship with him. I don't think about it. I'm not afraid of getting AIDS. I probably should be more worried, but what good will that do?"

Commentary

Given the danger of transmitting HIV disease, the participants asked if they should be sexual with other people at all. They craved involvement with individuals who would provide comfort and meaning for them and help to meet their sexual needs. As Marilyn put it, "I long for a companion to love me, AIDS and all. Because of AIDS, I may have to live without a companion."

However, the PWAs did not want to infect anyone, and the significant persons feared becoming infected themselves. Roxanne said, "I don't want to be the cause of somebody dying, because life is precious." They questioned whether using condoms would, in fact, prohibit HIV transmission. "I take precautions to not infect my wife," Tonio said, "but I'm concerned that they will not work." In asking whether they should be sexual, the participants expressed concern about AIDS taking away their sexuality. Bruce asked, "How should I deal with the unfairness of AIDS and its effect on my sexuality?"

Most participants resolved their conflict by being sexual. Jacob and Diana said that they only engaged in sex with other HIV-infected individuals. As Jacob put it, "To be fair, I want to be involved with someone who's also infected so I don't infect anyone else. An infected person will know what AIDS is like."

The PWAs who were sexual described a second conflict, whether to tell their potential sexual partners about having AIDS. On one hand, they said that HIV-infected persons should be honest about their diagnosis. As Vance explained, "It is unethical to have sex, even if it is protected sex, without telling her that I have AIDS."

On the other hand, the PWAs were reluctant to be honest with their sexual partners because they feared rejection. Also, they were angry about their diagnosis and being stigmatized by society. Roxanne said, "A lot of people think somebody gave them AIDS, and they're going to give it to everybody."

Many of the PWAs acknowledged that they had engaged in sex without disclosing their diagnosis or using protection, particularly right after being diagnosed with HIV infection. "When I was diagnosed," explained Bruce, "I wanted to share HIV with everybody. I had unsafe, casual sex." The participants described a third conflict. Even if they decided to be sexual and talk openly about HIV disease, they questioned whether to use condoms. The women hesitated to ask their male sexual partners to use condoms. As Marilyn put it, "He may reject me if I insist on condoms." Shari said, "He refuses to use condoms, and I'm afraid I will become infected. He's more comfortable without condoms. All men are like that."

The women worried that if they did not sexually satisfy their partners, the men would be promiscuous or reject them and even transmit HIV disease to someone else. Diana, who felt too sick to have sex, said, "My boyfriend is a man and I can't expect him not to have sex because I don't have sex. I'm worried about my boyfriend passing HIV to somebody. He gave HIV to me." Margo explained about her husband who had AIDS, "My husband has a high sex drive. When a man is not satisfied, he's going to go somewhere else and get it. I rather him stay here and get sex."

The men explained that condoms reduced their sexual satisfaction and could lead to sexual impotence. Some male PWAs even said that if their sexual partners were willing, they did not use condoms. "The ones that wanted a condom," said Andy, "didn't make a difference to me. I felt that we can do this to keep you safe." However, he acknowledged, "With my present girlfriend, sometimes we use condoms, and sometimes we don't, the emotion at the moment." His girlfriend, Shari, said, "For the first 6 months we were together, I didn't know he's infected, and we didn't use condoms. I found out by overhearing him on the phone, and I cried. I don't want to get AIDS because I have children. One is disabled."

Even if the participants had engaged in unsafe sex in the past, most of them said that now they were taking steps to avoid HIV transmission, primarily through celibacy, being honest about AIDS, and using protection when engaging in sex. Jacob explained, "If you're a sexually responsible person, you protect yourself and the other person."

Some participants said that because of AIDS they were changing their views about sexuality. "I am a sexual person through nurturing, love, respect, and sharing," Eric said, describing his new perspective. "Sex doesn't need a nasty element to be fun. Sex isn't bad, it's a wonderful gift." Martin said, "From my relationship with my lover, I'm learning that sexuality and sexual intercourse aren't the same. I have to be myself, doing what feels good, safe, responsible."

Despite AIDS, some participants said that they were able to meet their sexual needs in caring relationships. "I am sexually active in my monogamous relationship," explained Eric. "I won't endanger my partner if I don't engage in activities that transmit HIV. HIV-infected persons build relationships that are loving with noninfected persons, and people start relationships with HIV-infected persons. They're having rich, full relationships."

The participants' stories support research findings indicating that HIV-infected persons frequently do not disclose their infection to their sexual partners (Marks, Richardson, & Maldonado, 1991; McCusker, Stoddard, & McCarthy, 1992; Schoeman, 1991). Persons with HIV disease who have been honest about their diagnosis have been subject to discrimination and ruptured relationships (Winslade, 1989). Individuals who knowingly expose other people to HIV disease may be reacting to their experience of discrimination, poverty, and alienation (Poku, 1992).

Research has documented inequities in power between some women and men, as illustrated by the participants' stories. Traditionally, women have assumed responsibility for using protection when engaging in sex. Often, they feel that they have little personal power to demand that men use condoms, and even think that HIV infection is their due (Bell, 1989).

Several studies have been reported about inconsistent use of condoms (Jemmott & Jemmott, 1991; Smeltzer & Whipple, 1991; Williams, 1991). Additional research is needed to identify what should be done to encourage women to insist on protection when engaging in sex even though they risk losing their male partners. Also, research is needed about how to encourage men to value their female sexual partners over their own sexual satisfaction and take responsibility for using safer sex techniques.

Codependency is one explanation for why a non-HIV-infected individual would knowingly engage in unprotected sex with someone who has HIV disease. Lisa, who used condoms "sometimes," said, "I'm fine having a sexual relationship with him. I don't think about it. I'm not afraid of getting AIDS." Shari explained, "If I wanted to use condoms, he'd be willing, but I don't want nothing to be uncomfortable for him. I think more of him than myself. He's not planning to be with a girl no more than a night or couple of days, but I take it one step at a time." A few months later, the nurse who had arranged my interview with Shari told me that she had become HIV-infected.

Codependency is extreme involvement with another person or persons, which can be so pervasive that the codependent's self-esteem depends on the other person. The individual feels unable to survive without the significant other. Codependency places the individual at risk for emotional, physical, and social difficulties, including HIV disease (St. Onge, 1992). Research is needed about effective ways to counteract codependency.

The participants' stories illustrate an important element that seems to be missing in current AIDS education. Being given information about AIDS does not appear to motivate some people to change their risky sexual behavior. Although all of the participants appeared to be knowledgeable about AIDS, some of them justified engaging in unsafe sexual practices. As Shari said, "It doesn't bother me that we don't use condoms because I go to the doctor regularly. If you're going to get AIDS, you're going to get AIDS. We all got to go some day."

The thinking of the participants who engaged in unsafe sex seemed to something like this: "Infecting another person or becoming infected is wrong, but being rejected is even worse. This one time I will engage in unprotected sex because the chance of the virus being transmitted is low." Research is needed to determine what kind of AIDS and ethics education are needed to overcome this type of reasoning so that people stop engaging in risky, unethical behavior while justifying their actions.

Gay PWAs described a fourth conflict involving sexuality. They questioned if they should hide being gay. As Tonio put it, "I lived most of my life feeling bad about being different. I tried to change so people would love me, but I couldn't change being gay. Should I be honest about who I am?" Tonio's words illustrate the struggle of many gay women and men to accept their sexuality in a homophobic world. Homophobia permeates society and the health care system (Crimp, 1988; Eliason & Randall, 1991). Repressive measures have been used to eliminate homosexual behavior and persons. Hatred and misunderstanding have been heaped upon homosexual women and men by their families, communities, government, organized religion, and even the gay community itself (Murphy, 1990, 1991a).

Because of homophobia, gay men have actually been blamed for AIDS. As Lewis put it, "People feel that if you weren't gay, AIDS wouldn't have happened." Some people have claimed that AIDS is a just punishment for homosexual behavior (Murphy, 1988).

Lewis and Theo described how they were dealing with homophobia. "When the voice inside says, 'If you hadn't been gay, you wouldn't have AIDS,' " said Lewis, "I answer with hope, strength, God. I say, 'I didn't choose to be gay. This is who I am.' " Theo explained, "I decided to love myself and be honest. Now I embrace my differences." He joined Alcoholics Anonymous, participated in the gay community, and became an AIDS activist.

Like Lewis and Theo, many gay, HIV-infected persons are coming to terms with their sexuality and refusing to internalize society's homophobia. They are avoiding abusive behavior, such as unsafe sex. Rather than be angry and depressed, they are using their struggles concerning sexuality as an opportunity for personal growth (Barrows & Halgin, 1988).

In summary, to deal effectively with AIDS, individuals need to take responsibility for their sexual behavior by not infecting anyone or becoming infected themselves. Society's responsibility is to fund research about sexuality, codependency, homophobia, and effective AIDS and ethics education and to provide education based on the findings.

14

The Basic Nature of Ethical Problems

The purpose of the research was to describe and examine the content and basic nature of PWAs' ethical problems. Chapters 4 to 13 address the content. In this chapter, I do a metaethical analysis to examine the basic nature of the participants' ethical problems and the ethical decision-making model that emerged. Each of the participants' ethical problems consisted of three components: conflict, resolution, and rationale. While discussing their ethical problems, the participants engaged in the three levels of ethical inquiry, addressed in Chapter 2. They did descriptive ethics and metaethics when they discussed their conflict, and they engaged in normative ethics and metaethics when they talked about their resolution to the conflict and their rationale for their resolution.

Certainly, these three components provide an understanding of the basic nature of PWAs' ethical problems involving AIDS. However, ethical problems experienced by PWAs may not be identical to ethical problems involving other phenomena. AIDS primarily affects young people, and it is life-threatening, contagious, chronic, and stigmatizing. The PWAs said that they felt pressure to resolve their ethical problems before dying. Even with these limitations, the components provide a starting point for understanding the basic nature of ethical problems in general.

Conflict (Descriptive Ethics and Metaethics)

The participants described their conflict as a clash of values about the right way to live and die in relation to other people. Three kinds of competing values were in conflict: (1) what to believe, (2) who to be, and (3) what to do. These kinds of values are related to the three components of Aristotle's (1987) virtue ethics, which consist of contemplative reasoning, moral virtue, and calculative reasoning.

One PWA, for example, said that he wanted to tell his extended family about his diagnosis. His parents, whom he loved, had asked him to keep his diagnosis, sexuality, and lover a secret. Because he hoped to live and die well, he questioned if he should believe that his first responsibility was to himself or his parents. Should he be honest or caring? Should he tell his extended family or not?

Because their conflict was stressful, the participants said that they felt pressure to resolve it as soon as possible. At the same time, they wanted to resolve it well so that they would feel good about themselves and their relationships. Most of them cried as they talked because of the pain that they were experiencing from their conflict.

In describing their conflict, most of the participants did not use the language of academic ethics, such as terms like *beneficence* and *justice.* However, all of them said that they wanted to determine what was the "right thing to do" about their conflict, whether or not they eventually did what they said that they should do. With everyday language, they talked about what was bothering them.

Ethical, theological, and psychological concerns were woven together. The participants did not separate their ethical concerns from other concerns. A PWA, for example, questioned whether he should commit suicide. He said, "I don't know how long I will live or what will happen to me after I die." He wondered if taking his life would ever be justifiable. Would God forgive him for ending his life? What was the right way to cope with his anxiety concerning these questions?

Conflict of one ethical problem overlapped with conflict of another ethical problem. Although I asked them to describe the ethical problem causing them the *most* conflict, each participant discussed several overlapping ethical problems. For example, a PWA asked if she should be sexual with a man, given the danger of infecting him with HIV disease. That conflict led to another conflict, whether she should risk rejection by telling him about her diagnosis and insisting on protection when engaging in sex.

For the participants, conflict was ongoing. Another ethical problem appeared as they resolved one ethical problem. For example, a PWA questioned whether she should tell people at work about her diagnosis. She told them during the 2 weeks between her first and second interviews. At the second interview, she said that as a result of being honest about her diagnosis, she now was confronted with discrimination at work. She described conflict about the right way to deal with this discrimination.

Apparent conflict covered hidden conflict. At the beginning of an interview, each participant described a common ethical problem, such as whether to use protection when engaging in sex. The person seemed to develop trust as the interview progressed and then talked about more personal, painful conflict. For example, a significant person questioned whether she should insist that her boyfriend wear condoms. She said, "My partner refuses to use condoms, but because all men are like that it doesn't bother me. It's not like he's going to be with anyone else." An hour later, she tearfully acknowledged that he was not monogamous although she was "risking my life for him."

Hidden conflict often consisted of complicated, painful questions about personhood. For example, a PWA described conflict concerning whether to use marijuana and LSD. The longer he talked, however, the more his conflict centered on what kind of person to be. Although he said that he had been given a religious education, he no longer went to church because he was an "agnostic." "If there is a God, why do I have AIDS?" he asked. "Should I believe in God in order to have the comfort of knowing that I will go to heaven when I die?"

Many participants expressed difficulty explaining why they felt conflict. While talking about their conflict during the first interview, they brought it into focus. At the second interview, they said the first interview and their reflection on it were helping them to understand their conflict. For example, a PWA said, "This process helped me to identify a problem and to consolidate things in my mind, to think about where I stand on the problem. I appreciate the chance to do this."

The PWAs and significant persons described similar conflict, except that for the most part, the PWAs focused on themselves but the significant persons focused on the PWAs. Possibly this difference resulted from the emphasis of the research on PWAs' ethical problems. For example, a PWA described conflict about whether he should give in to despair about his deteriorating health or live as fully as possible, whereas his mother described conflict about whether she should give in to despair about her son's deteriorating health or live as fully as possible.

The conflict of the PWAs and significant persons differed in yet another significant way. The PWAs could not run away from AIDS. In contrast, the significant persons had some choice about whether to stay with or leave the PWAs, and they agonized about the right thing to do.

Resolution (Normative Ethics and Metaethics)

The second component of the participants' ethical problems was resolution, what they said was the "right thing to do" about their conflict. Of the three kinds of normative ethical theories described in Chapter 2, virtue ethics (Aristotle, 1987) most resembles the participants' ethical decision-making process, although they took into account some aspects of principled thinking and ethical caring. Their resolutions were based on their beliefs (contemplative reasoning), desire to be a good person (moral virtue), and rational choice (calculative reasoning).

Identifying their beliefs was part of developing effective resolutions to their conflict. The participants described what they meant by beliefs. For example, a PWA said, "You instinctively know if you do something wrong." Another PWA said, "You never know what is the right thing, but I go by feeling and instinct, my internal values."

In response to AIDS, many of the participants were determining which beliefs were most important so that they could develop resolutions based on these beliefs. For example, a PWA said, "I have become less materialistic. I will work to make a living, but it's not as important now. It's more important that I have good friendships." Another PWA said, "I thought life was a big game. Life is about peace, love, and happiness. Everybody should be taking care of everybody else because they're lucky that they're alive. Because of AIDS, I see what life is really about." A significant person said, "I give greater value to intimacy, love, trust, relationships, life. I try to be more understanding of other people."

Besides beliefs, the participants based their resolutions on their desire to be a good person. For example, a significant person said, "Being a good person is right for me. Right means what is my nature, what's comfortable for me. This doesn't mean that it's right for someone else. It comes from inside of me and isn't imposed from the outside."

Basing their resolutions, in part, on the desire to be a good person had some similarities to ethical caring. The participants said that they were concerned about being compassionate. For example, a PWA said, "I am trying to be a good person who is loving, honest, hospitable, independent, hardworking, self-sufficient."

Finally, in addition to their beliefs and desire to be a good person, the participants took into account rational choice when developing resolutions to their conflict. They tried to step back from their particular situation and see it more objectively in order to make a good decision about the right way to resolve their conflict. This part of their ethical decision-making process had some similarities to principled thinking.

As part of rational choice, the participants tried to balance deontology (right action) and consequentialism (good consequences). For example, a PWA said, "The right way to live is to treat everybody fair. Don't offend God, other people, yourself. Don't steal, don't tell a lie." Another PWA said, "I try not to hurt anybody, and if I can do something good for someone, I do it. I try to live by the Golden Rule, treat people as you want them to treat you." To avoid discrimination, a PWA had lied to a co-worker about AIDS medications. He explained, "I don't feel good about lying but it's more important not to hurt myself than to tell a white lie. There's that balance thing." Not all of the participants' resolutions were based on a combination of their beliefs, desire to be a good person, and rational choice. Often, they described how they ideally wanted to resolve their ethical problems, not how they actually resolved them. For example, a PWA said, "If I didn't have HIV, I wouldn't want nobody giving it to me. You might be taking a life, and that's wrong." However, he later admitted, "With my present girlfriend, sometimes we use condoms, and sometimes we don't, the emotion at the moment." His girlfriend said that they engaged in unsafe sex because he refused to wear condoms. A few months after her interviews, she was diagnosed with HIV disease herself.

Another PWA explained that she wanted to be a good mother. Later, she acknowledged that she would continue to inject drugs that she said were not good for her or her children. A third PWA told about volunteering as an AIDS educator because he was concerned about ethical problems. Yet, he said that he secretly used illegal drugs, did not consistently use condoms, and told his girlfriend that he was monogamous although he engaged in unsafe sex with other women.

Rationale (Normative Ethics and Metaethics)

The third component of the participants' ethical problems was rationale, their explanations for their resolutions. They said that "right resolutions" helped them to live with meaning, which in general meant seeing their life as part of a bigger, purposeful picture. A significant person, for example, explained why she had decided to stay in a sexual relationship with her boyfriend who had AIDS. She said, "Part of the purpose of life is to make life better, and we make each other's lives better. He encourages me to get over my shyness, and I help him with a positive attitude."

Moreover, the participants explained that "right resolutions" helped them to behave with integrity, which in general they defined as living according to their beliefs. For example, a PWA said,

"To feel good about myself, I try to be a nice person who is unselfish." A significant person said, "What's morally right is to help other people first. I want to act in such a way that I am not in conflict with myself." When talking about meaning and integrity, some participants used the word *spirituality*. For them, spirituality meant harmony with the whole of things, which was not necessarily the same as belief in God or adherence to organized religion. For example, a PWA explained, "Being spiritual means realizing that I have an inner power which guides me and holds the mysteries of wonder, life, and change. I can be spiritual and pray without going to church and subscribing to dogma."

For some participants, their belief in God helped them to live with meaning and integrity. For example, a PWA said, "God as you understand Him will come into your life to let you realize His will be done. Different things are put in people's lives to let them see that there's something more than what we know to make life worth living." Another PWA said, "If I didn't have God to trust in, I'd have a difficult time." A significant person said, "You cling to what is true and real, what you live by, who you are. These solid values became important, values of family, friendships, faith in God, love for each other. We let slide other things such as social living, money, entertainment."

Some participants explained that being involved with organized religion resulted in meaning and integrity. For example, a PWA said that he had converted to Roman Catholicism after nearly dying. Since then, he had been trying to lead his life according to those religious values.

For the participants, choosing to live with meaning and integrity helped create "harmony out of chaos," provided an explanation for suffering, and guided them in resolving their ethical problems. Then they did not feel as alone, and they were not as afraid of death. As they habituated themselves to ethical living, they no longer experienced as many ethical problems, such as whether to engage in unsafe sex. For example, a PWA said, "Being on my spiritual, healing journey resolves many ethical problems for me. I don't have many ethical problems anymore."

The participants varied in the degree to which they were experiencing meaning and integrity. Some of them described feeling victimized, alienated, and powerless. Others talked about living with meaning and integrity despite deteriorating health. For example, a PWA said, "My being gay and having AIDS has enriched my life." Another PWA said, "I'm grateful to AIDS for opening my sense of empowerment. AIDS is a gift."

Many participants admitted that at times they knowingly had resolved their conflict in what they referred to as a "wrong way," such as neglecting to use protection while having sex. They did not clearly answer the age-old question: Why do people knowingly engage in what they say is wrong behavior? Their thinking seemed to be something like this: "In general, such an action is wrong. At the moment of the action, however, I did not think that the action was wrong for me because of extenuating circumstances, such as my legitimate fear of rejection or the momentary pleasure I would receive from the activity."

How the participants defined right and wrong differed considerably. For example, a PWA who was a former bank robber justified robbing banks to obtain money for heroin and cocaine. He said, "Bankers are rich and should share" and "my gun was not loaded." He said that he no longer robbed banks because he did not want to go back to prison. Without money from bank robberies, he could not afford to buy drugs, and he was sober.

In contrast, several PWAs became AIDS activists because "it was the right thing to do." They said that they wanted to help educate other people about ethics and AIDS, which included living by ethical values themselves. Explaining why he became an AIDS activist, a PWA said, "Helping other people helps me feel better about myself." Another PWA justified being an AIDS activist, even though it brought stress into his life. "I've survived so long with AIDS because of my activism," he said.

While explaining their rationale, the participants expressed doubt, as if they were seeking reassurance that they were "doing the right thing" about their conflict. They were critical of themselves, explaining that they were not living up to their values. They eloquently described the universal human struggle to live in the right way with some feeling of security in the midst of unpredictability.

An Ethical Decision-Making Model

Chapter 2 includes a brief description of ethical decision-making models that have been developed to help resolve ethical problems (Beauchamp & Childress, 1989; Cameron & Schaffer, 1991; Frankena, 1973; Thiroux, 1986). Many clinicians appreciate an ethical decision-making model, which can be used to identify ethical components, provide a framework for developing a resolution, and furnish language that facilitates discussion and brings together heterogeneous individuals.

Although the models described in Chapter 2 may be helpful, the participants' method of ethical decision making suggests that models not taking into account beliefs, character, and rational choice are inadequate. A comprehensive, yet easily understood, ethical decision-making model emerged from the participants' stories. The model consists of three steps: (1) What should I believe? (2) Who should I be? and (3) What should I do? These steps, summarized in Figure 14.1, are similar to virtue ethics (Aristotle, 1987), consisting of contemplative reasoning, moral virtue, and calculative reasoning. To resolve an ethical problem using this model, an individual would develop responses to the three questions.

Answering the first question (What should I believe?) necessitates engaging in contemplative reasoning. Ideally, a person would ask this question throughout life, not just at the time of experiencing a particular ethical problem, and would develop beliefs that provide meaning. For Aristotle (1987), the object of contemplative reasoning was an "intuitive grasp of first principles." He did not elaborate on what he meant by this concept, but it may be similar to an "ah-hah experience" that one can have when looking at a beautiful scene, reading thought-provoking literature, watching a baby being born, and being at someone's deathbed. At that moment, one might say, "Now I know what life is about."

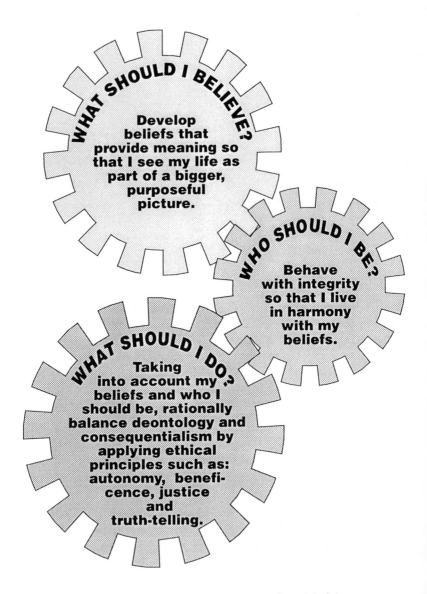

Figure 14.1. Research-Based Ethical Decision-Making Model

To answer the second question (Who should I be?), ideally an individual would develop moral virtue, or excellent character, on an ongoing basis, rather than confront the question for the first time when experiencing a specific ethical problem. Day in and day out, the person habitually would behave with integrity by living in harmony with the beliefs identified in question one. Part of being a good person is to be caring (Noddings, 1984). Aristotle (1987) defined excellent character as a disposition to be moderate, rather than excessive, in one's behavior.

An individual would answer the third question (What should I do?) when confronted with a particular ethical problem. Taking into account answers to the first two questions, the person would engage in calculative reasoning. An effective way to balance deontological concerns (right actions) and consequentialist concerns (good consequences) is by applying appropriate ethical principles, such as autonomy, beneficence, justice, and truth-telling. After prioritizing these principles according their importance, the person would logically develop a resolution that leads to meaning and integrity.

This model can be used to resolve ethical problems on individual, institutional, professional, and societal levels. Many persons may be involved with a particular ethical problem, such as the right way to allocate scarce health care resources. In this case, members of the group would individually answer the first two questions. Then working together they would rationally develop a resolution in response to the third question. Ideally, the resolution would eliminate the problem, while facilitating each person involved to live with meaning and integrity.

In summary, the ethical decision-making model that emerged from the research may be more reflective of human behavior than current models in use because it takes into account individual beliefs, desire to be a good person, and rational choice. Additional empirical research and philosophical analysis are needed to develop effective ethical decision-making models.

15

Ethical Living

Human beings experience ethical problems. On a daily basis, age-old questions clamor for answers: What should I believe? Who should I be? What should I do? By drawing on philosophical ethics and the participants' experience, this book provides assistance for conceptualizing and resolving ethical problems.

Besides questioning how to live ethically, many of us wonder about the right way to help other people who are experiencing painful ethical problems. As nurses, physicians, therapists, teachers, and friends, we want to assist our clients and loved ones to resolve what is bothering them. The participants' stories suggest strategies for facilitating ethical living.

Ethical Beliefs, Character, and Actions

One strategy is to develop ethical beliefs and an ethical character, and to act ethically. Ethical beliefs provide meaning to life. In general, the participants defined *meaning* as seeing their life as part of a bigger, purposeful picture. Their stories provide examples of beliefs, the most common of which was belief in an underlying order. Engaging in what Aristotle (1987) referred to as contemplative reasoning, they developed ethical beliefs by meditating, reading thought-provoking literature, listening to music, being present at someone's deathbed, and discussing ethical problems with friends. Some of the participants said that organized religion helped them, whereas other participants turned to support groups. Ethical character, or excellent disposition, means to be a good person. According to the participants, a good person consistently behaves with integrity, which in general they defined as living in harmony with one's ethical beliefs. They expressed concern about being a good person, not a bad one. Some of the characteristics that they used to describe a good person were "loving, honest, hospitable, independent, hardworking, self-sufficient, trusting, polite, unselfish, and nice." A good person was "accepting and kept going, instead of being angry and giving up." Rather than "trying to control everything," a good person acknowledged personal "powerlessness."

Ethical actions result from what Aristotle (1987) called calculative reasoning, which takes into account ethical beliefs and character. The participants talked about making rational, responsible choices concerning their actions. For the most part, they said that they did not want to hurt anyone, and if possible, they wanted to help instead. To determine which actions were ethical, they tried to balance deontological concerns (right actions) and consequentialist concerns (good consequences). An ethical decision-making model can be helpful for determining which actions are ethical (Beauchamp & Childress, 1989; Cameron & Schaffer, 1992; Frankena, 1973; Thiroux, 1986).

Ethical beliefs, character, and actions can enable an individual to live ethically in a complicated world that includes HIV disease. In short, this ethic consists of behaving responsibly toward oneself and other people. Certainly, responsible behavior means to choose actions that neither transmit HIV infection to another person nor allow oneself to become HIV-infected (Bateson & Goldsby, 1988).

Some people may think that they lack the resources and freedom to live ethically. For example, they may know that their actions put them at risk for HIV disease, but they are locked into dangerous patterns, such as abusive sexual behavior. They may be facing a slow, painful death or love someone who is near death. Yet they can make responsible choices leading to meaning and integrity (Bateson & Goldsby, 1988).

Ethics Education

A second strategy for facilitating ethical living is to learn more about ethical problems and how to resolve them. Some ways to become educated about ethics are by reading books on the topic, taking ethics classes, traveling, and learning about other cultures. An education in ethics provides philosophical tools for resolving ethical problems, which can enhance life.

Although anyone could benefit from a better understanding of ethics, the participants' stories suggest the need for health care personnel, in particular, to learn about ethical decision making. For example, a PWA who was a nurse said, "If we want to hold professionals accountable for making ethical decisions, that should be addressed in education." Increased ethical sensitivity can help health care personnel to avoid aggravating ethical problems or creating additional ethical problems for clients and themselves (Flack & Pellegrino, 1992; Matens, 1991).

The participants' stories suggest that ethics educators should include content about virtue ethics, meaning, and integrity in what they write or present. Life having meaning and behaving with integrity are not central to contemporary academic ethics (Wiggins, 1987), although a few philosophers have done work in the area (Dahl, 1987). Recently, some authors have suggested that ethics educators need to return to beneficence and virtue instead of focusing almost exclusively on rational thought (Cooper, 1990; Pellegrino & Thomasma, 1988).

Aristotle (1987) argued against circular thinking in which experience dictates values which dictate experience. He favored contemplative reasoning to "intuitively grasp first principles." With resulting philosophic wisdom, one engages in calculative reasoning in connection with moral virtue (excellent character) to resolve ethical problems. From this perspective, ethics educators who do not include contemplative reasoning, moral virtue, and calculative reasoning do not account for human beings' deep yearning for meaning and integrity.

Twenty-five hundred years ago, Aristotle's teacher, Plato (1961), wrote the *Symposium*. In it, Plato identified *eros* as the universal human response to self-conscious recognition of mortality. Human beings realize that they are in the inexorable process of dying. Eros is the effort to invest the transient, particular self with something beyond that has permanent, transcendent meaning. Facing unpredictability and death, the PWAs' desire for meaning and integrity was pronounced.

To apply the results of this research, effective ethics educators would include content about virtue ethics, meaning, and integrity, in addition to discussions of principled thinking and ethical caring. Coles (1989), a child psychiatrist who has conducted ethics research, concluded that ethical understanding comes not so much from scenarios postulated by theories as from literature, religion, and learning by example. Rather than focus on intellectual discussions about hypothetical problems, ethics educators would use examples from literature, diverse cultures, and stories of real people that elicit intuitive, compassionate responses in learners (Callahan, 1990; Campbell, 1990; Flack & Pellegrino, 1992; Matens, 1991; Younger, 1990).

Ethical Listening

A third strategy for facilitating ethical living is to engage in ethical listening. A serendipitous finding of the research was the importance of ethical listening. I used ethical listening to encourage the participants to describe their ethical problems. Besides benefiting the research, ethical listening proved to be a powerful independent intervention for helping the participants to resolve their ethical problems.

Ethical listening means actively and selectively focusing on a person's ethical conflict, instead of other subjects such as details about symptoms, medications, or treatments. The listener uses communication techniques such as "Go on" and "Tell me more" to encourage a complete description of the ethical problem. Rather than offer advice, the listener helps the person to articulate her or his own sense of the right thing to do about the ethical conflict so as to live with meaning and integrity.

The participants' stories suggest that ethics educators need to teach ethical listening to their students. Learning how to listen ethically requires knowledge about both ethical problems and communication techniques. By listening ethically, a person may be able to help a client, friend, family member, or someone else to effectively resolve an ethical problem.

Health care personnel, in particular, would benefit from learning how to engage in ethical listening. In fact, listening ethically may be the most important independent intervention that health care personnel can use to help their clients who are experiencing painful ethical problems. Each participant specifically mentioned how beneficial this kind of listening was.

"You are good listener," said a PWA. "Talking really helped. God bless you." Another PWA said, "I'd like to thank you for the opportunity to talk with you. This has added to my self-concept." A PWA wrote, "Thank you for including me in your study. I enjoyed the interview and especially your followup questions. Your unique ability to ask good questions has not been experienced by me in other interviews that I've had." A significant person said, "It's been a pleasure; you draw me out."

The participants explained that ethical listening helped them to resolve their ethical problems. For example, one PWA, who had become HIV-infected from a blood transfusion to treat his hemophilia, asked, "Is it right to be prejudiced toward the gay community? I am bitter because the chance that one of them gave blood that infected me is pretty good." After talking through his ethical problem, he said, "I don't think it's right to be prejudiced towards anyone for any reason. This last 30 seconds I've come about as close as I ever have to resolving this ethical problem, although I don't know if I'll ever resolve it."

Another PWA explained how ethical listening had benefited him. "This process helped me identify a problem and to consolidate things in my mind," he said, "to think about where I stand on the problem. I appreciate the chance to do this."

Yet another PWA said that talking was so useful that he was going to see a counselor. "Never have I been interviewed in such a thorough, sensitive manner," he said. "It helped me clarify my thinking. I will give the counselor a copy of the analysis."

At the second interview, I gave each participant my written analysis of the first interview. Reading the analysis seemed therapeutic. For example, at the first interview, a significant person described why she engaged in unprotected sex with her boyfriend who had AIDS, even though she was afraid of becoming HIV-infected. As she read the analysis she said, "Looks harder written down than when you think about it. You want to cry."

The participants expressed a longing for health care personnel to engage in ethical listening with them. They said that health care personnel for the most part focus on diet, medications, treatments, appointments, and other concrete issues, but do not ask about clients' experiences. For example, a PWA said, "It's wonderful that your study looks at the viewpoints from a PWA perspective as opposed to the clinician's views."

If health care personnel are provided with appropriate education about ethics and communication techniques, they will be able to engage in ethical listening with their clients. For example, a nurse could listen ethically while doing daily cares for a client. A physician could engage in ethical listening during an office call.

Ethical listening by health care personnel can assist clients to resolve their ethical problems. With the knowledge gained through ethical listening, health care personnel would be more effective advocates for clients. An understanding of ethical problems experienced by clients could even help health care personnel to resolve their own ethical problems involving health care. Health care personnel who engage in effective ethical listening will be able to provide more knowledgeable care for clients and enhance their health-related outcomes.

Ethical Society

A fourth strategy for facilitating ethical living is to work for a more ethical society in which the kinds of ethical problems described by the participants are less likely to occur. Ethical living not only results from individuals making responsible choices about their own behavior. Society also has responsibility to help people live with meaning and integrity. According to many of the participants, individuals who desire to live ethically have a mandate to work for a more ethical society. For example, a PWA explained why he had chosen to be a nurse and an AIDS activist. "A sense of integrity comes," he said, "provided I take care of myself. Helping other people enhances the quality of my life by giving me purpose, meaning, satisfaction. We have gross ethical inequities in the system, and I'm going to do what I can to make things better."

An ethical society directly addresses the kinds of ethical problems described by the participants, whether these problems involve alcohol and drugs, chronic illness, death, discrimination, finances and business, health care, personhood, relationships, service, or sexuality (Bayer, 1991b; Daniels, 1992; Fox, 1987; Fowler, 1988a; Funkhouser & Moser, 1990). In an ethical society, public policy concerning AIDS or any other issue does not result from stereotypes or punitive attitudes. Instead, the government and private sector work together to fund research so that public policy is based on knowledge (Gaskins, Sowell, & Gueldner, 1991).

A major theme arising from the participants' stories is the importance of more research. Both quantitative and qualitative methodologies can provide better understanding of society's ethical problems and how to best resolve them (Cooper & Weiss, 1989; C. Levine, 1991). Research is needed to develop effective answers to ethical problems such as: How should individual autonomy and communitarian values be balanced (Nelkin et al., 1990)? What is quality health care, and how should it be provided in an economical, efficient, and caring manner? What is the right way to promote individual responsibility (Bayer, 1992)?

Society has choices, just as individuals do. As members of society, we can view ethical problems as an opportunity to improve ourselves and society or as a source of despair and alienation. When confronted by ethical problems, we can creatively resolve them, or we can angrily lash out at other imperfect human beings. We can open doors, or we can slam doors shut (Nelkin et al., 1990).

During the Second World War, individuals living in the small French Protestant village of Le Chambon risked their lives to save about 6,000 people, most of them Jews, from the Nazis. When later asked why they had helped, they answered, "There was nothing else to do." Assisting other human beings whom society had rejected but who were desperately in need of help was for them as natural as breathing or eating. In the ethical climate that the villagers had created, they viewed what they had done as necessary, not praiseworthy (Hallie, 1989). An ethical society produces people like those villagers. Instead of turning away from PWAs and other people in need, we step forward and offer to help.

APPENDIX

A Transcriber's Experience

After completing the interviews, I interviewed the transcriber of the audiotapes for 25 of the 30 participants. She discussed how her experience with the research was affecting her view of the participants, AIDS, and ethics. Her struggle to verbalize her reactions may help you to put into words your own responses to the participants' stories.

Participants

"When you're plugged into the dictation equipment, you are living somebody else's experience. You hear if they hurt or don't hurt and they're happy or sad. I wanted to tell somebody, but I couldn't because of confidentiality. I had to transcribe the tapes during the day, or I couldn't sleep. What they said kept recycling through my head. It was better for me to quit a good hour before I went to bed.

"I felt like I got to know them as persons because they really opened up. Particularly those who were concerned about confidentiality. They said things that they couldn't say any place else. How often does anybody get to sit and chat one to one for an hour about their deepest inner concerns? Some of what they said may have been for shock value, but I think they were telling the truth. I don't think anybody lied.

"The beginning of each interview was more superficial. For every person, the deepest, darkest parts came spilling out at the end. By then, they felt comfortable and weren't going to stop talking until they got it out. There seemed to be a certain point, for some it took longer than others, where they reached in, grabbed you and said, 'This is what I really mean.' They were trying to describe a little piece of what life was like for them. Their inner feelings, how they saw it, how they felt about it. That's a tough thing for people to do.

"They opened up when they had enough trust. The questions encouraged them to go deeper. It takes a while to get it all together in your head. Yes, they knew the interviews were coming. Certainly their lives were threatened, but I don't think they could say that right up front. The settings helped them to talk. It was quiet and one on one, and there wasn't outside interference. At some point, they forgot the tape was running, and they were more expressive. Maybe at the end they were looking for help, a little guidance.

"In other research I've transcribed, the interviews were done in 20 or 30 minutes. They were looking for easier things. What's it like to live here? There are many ways to answer that, and everybody took the easiest route. People said what was conventional, expected. Maybe in 60 minutes somebody would have said, 'I hate it here!' But in 30 minutes they didn't. People aren't going to automatically talk about that in the first few minutes. You have to go to depths and get at people's values for them to give their own unique perception of life. What it is for them personally."

AIDS

"Each participant touches your inner part. It's so sad. They're probably going to die young, and it's not pleasant. 'My friends deserted me because I have AIDS. I'm going to die alone, and when I'm dead nobody's going to mourn my loss.' Hearing them talk wasn't like watching TV or a movie. It was a whole different thing.

"If my job consisted of listening to that every day, I couldn't stay cued in enough to let them express themselves. There is a point where the wall goes up, the door slams shut. I don't want to think that everybody is dying of AIDS. How could you listen for 8 hours and keep your sense of balance, or not think that life is very sad?

"For me, the most heartbreaking participants were the gay men. The whole gay community seems to be shunned, and the participants certainly were. It seems like a sad life-style. Yet, when they're close to somebody, it's just as rewarding a relationship as for any heterosexual. That was uplifting.

"I developed a relationship with the man who didn't go to his class reunion because he didn't want the people in his home town to know that he had AIDS. I cried because I felt bad for him. He probably would have gotten compassion from his former classmates, but he cut it off. My tears were about him feeling alone in the world, the ultimate loneliness. We could probably all be there.

"Can you imagine having the secret about AIDS bottled up inside of you, forever, it must seem like? If you keep it inside, you can feel your stomach twist. And to live day after day with that constant twisting going on because you can't dump it some place must be horrible. And some of them do that. Yet, they may be right to keep AIDS a secret if people hold it against them. Maybe this is the only way they can exist. But I think the ones who get support are better off.

"The interviews have given me better understanding of people with AIDS. As I listened to the drug users, it seemed like there was much more involved in why they were doing drugs. That somehow JUST SAY NO doesn't make it go away. But maybe that's a start. Before, if I knew someone with AIDS, I might have said, 'I'm sorry to hear that,' and go about my business. Now I would be more attentive because most of them are very much alone and cut off, and maybe they need to talk."

Ethics

"The interviews have been an ethics education because they have made me think about who I am as a person. They haven't changed my values, but they have helped to define them. I've learned that people's values differ.

"I've always thought, 'Is this something I should do or not?' But now it's become ethical and not ethical. When you put it in that context, it's a more important issue, no matter how small. It's a matter of where you draw the line. The interviews have made me more aware of where my line is.

"Is what some of them did any worse than something I have done? The pens that were in my kitchen belong to the company I work for. I didn't think of myself as a thief because having them wasn't hurting anybody. But those pens weren't mine. The company didn't owe them to me. So I brought them back. The interviews make you think. Do I follow my own value system? Am I even aware of what I'm doing?

"Why did I bring the pens back? It was the right thing to do. That made me feel better. Nobody would find them or even care. It only had to do with my inner self and feeling right about who I am. When it feels OK inside, I know. I also know when it doesn't feel good, and I don't like that. Some of it comes with us, but I also think that it's taught. Maybe the person has the potential as a child, but through the right education the child learns.

"Behaving with integrity is the only way for me to live. Once you realize that what you have done is not right, you have to make amends so that you can wake up the next morning and comb your hair and look in the mirror and feel good about yourself and go to work. In the case of the guys who can't make amends for transmitting HIV, that's a situation I don't ever want to be in. The damage is done, and it's irretrievable. If I couldn't take it back, it would be difficult to live with myself. I wouldn't be able to die a peaceful death. I want to die knowing that I didn't do any great harm and, hopefully, did some good.

"My tears are related to the man who died after his third interview. He died a good death, the way I want to die. His lover and his family cared for him. He knew that he was leaving them behind, and that's tough. He was younger than me. Maybe the tears have to do with knowing that I'll be there some day. The emotional impact of talking to people who are facing death. When they shouldn't be. And feeling sad.

"A lot of life is luck. So many things can happen and don't by a split second. You weren't at that intersection at that particular time, or you weren't with that HIV-infected person. But you could have been. You're one breath away from being in their shoes. What gives him the path that he has taken and me the path that I have taken?

"I can't sit in judgment of the participants. Even the IV [intravenous] drug users who are into stealing and prostitution. If I were in their situation, maybe I'd do the same thing. What is their background? Why are they where they're at? What was

different in their life that got them to that point and didn't get me to
that point?

"The participants' stories had more of an impact on me than if
I'd read a paper about being sensitive to people with AIDS. It's
somebody's real life. Stories communicate on a deeper level because that person is a lot like me. Hearing people's stories and
talking about them helps put things in place. Otherwise, it's this
swirling thing, and you think, 'What is the point?' Talking about
their stories gives meaning to them. I need meaning, rather than just,
'Why did this happen?' I need to know how it fits with my life.

"The interviews get at my deep, unanswered questions: Why
am I here? Where am I going? Why do they have AIDS, and I
don't? The interviews don't give answers. There aren't right answers. There are things that you can't control. How can I lead a
meaningful life with this unpredictability?

"The tears are because I wonder if I'm a good person. Will I
make the right choices, do the right thing? Maybe I'll end up like
the participants, and I can't get myself out of it. I have to make
decisions without knowing how they'll come out, and it's only
later that I'll be able to say, 'I did well' or 'I messed up.' If my
choices only affected me, it would be easier, but they impact other
people's lives.

"I don't think it's clear what kind of person to be. So I want to
act without regrets. To feel like a good person. Persons with AIDS
don't have as many options as I do. I can't look to my family or
my work situation for what makes my life meaningful. I get
satisfaction from what's inside of me. I like somebody to say, 'You
did a nice job' or 'You can always count on her because she'll do
it right.' That helps me achieve. But in the end, it's what's inside."

References

Ackerman, S. J. (1990). Health-care workers take AIDS in stride. *The Journal of NIH Research, 2,* 30-31.

Ackiron, E. (1991). Patents for critical pharmaceuticals: The AZT case. *American Journal of Law and Medicine, 17,* 145-180.

Adair, M. N., Nygard, N. K., Maddox, R. W., & Adair, J. B. (1991). New behavioral strategies for enhancing immune function. *AIDS Patient Care, 5,* 297-300.

Adler, M. W. (1991). HIV, confidentiality and a "delicate balance." *Journal of Medical Ethics, 17,* 196-198.

Alexander, R., & Fitzpatrick, J. (1991). Variables influencing nurses' attitudes toward AIDS and AIDS patients. *AIDS Patient Care, 5,* 315-320.

Allen, D. M., Onorato, I. M., Green, T. A., & the Field Services Branch of the Centers for Disease Control. (1992). HIV infection in intravenous drug users entering drug treatment, United States, 1988 to 1989. *American Journal of Public Health, 82,* 541-546.

Allers, C. T. (1990). AIDS and the older adult. *The Gerontologist, 30,* 405-407.

Almond, B., & Ulanowsky, C. (1990). HIV and pregnancy. *Hastings Center Report, 20*(2), 16-21.

American Nurses Association. (1985). *Code for nurses with interpretive statements.* Kansas City, MO: Author.

American Nurses Association. (1991). *Nursing's agenda for health care reform.* Kansas City, MO: Author.

American Nurses Association. (1992). *Compendium of HIV/AIDS positions, policies and documents.* Washington, DC: Author.

ANA Committee on Ethics. (1988). *Statement regarding risk versus responsibility in providing nursing care.* Kansas City, MO: American Nurses Association.

Anderson, J. M. (1990). Home care management in chronic illness and the self-care movement. *Advances in Nursing Science, 12*(2), 71-83.

Aristotle. (1987). *The Nicomachean ethics* (D. Ross, Trans., 1954; J. L. Ackrill & J. O. Urmson, Revisors, 1973). New York: Oxford University Press.

229

Armstrong-Esther, C., & Hewitt, W. E. (1990). The effect of education on nurses' perception of AIDS. *Journal of Advanced Nursing, 15,* 638-651.

Arras, J. D. (1990). Noncompliance in AIDS research. *Hastings Center Report, 20*(5), 24-32.

Ashery, R. S. (1992). Issues in AIDS training for substance abuse workers. *Journal of Substance Abuse Treatment, 9,* 15-19.

Barbacci, M., Repke, J. T., & Chaisson, R. E. (1991). Routine prenatal screening for HIV infection. *Lancet, 337,* 709-711.

Barrows, P. A., & Halgin, R. P. (1988). Current issues in psychotherapy with gay men. *Professional Psychology: Research and Practice, 19,* 395-402.

Bateson, M. C., & Goldsby, R. (1988). *Thinking AIDS.* Reading, MA: Addison-Wesley.

Battin, M. P. (1992). Assisted suicide: Can we learn from Germany? *Hastings Center Report, 22*(2), 44-51.

Bayer, R. (1989). *Private acts, social consequences.* New York: Free Press.

Bayer, R. (1990). AIDS and the future of reproductive freedom. *The Milbank Quarterly, 68,* 179-204.

Bayer, R. (1991a). Introduction: The great drug policy debate—What means this thing called decriminalization? *The Milbank Quarterly, 69,* 341-363.

Bayer, R. (1991b). Public health policy and the AIDS epidemic: An end to HIV exceptionalism? *New England Journal of Medicine, 324,* 1500-1504.

Bayer, R. (1992). AIDS and liberalism: A response to Patricia Illingworth. *Bioethics, 6*(1), 23-27.

Beauchamp, T. L., & Childress, J. F. (1989). *Principles of biomedical ethics* (3rd ed.). New York: Oxford University Press.

Bell, N. K. (1989). Women and AIDS: Too little, too late? *Hypatia, 4*(3), 3-22.

Bell, N. K. (1991). Ethical issues in AIDS education. In F. G. Reamer (Ed.), *AIDS & ethics* (pp. 128-154). New York: Columbia University Press.

Benjamin, A. E. (1988). Long-term care and AIDS. *The Milbank Quarterly, 66,* 415-443.

Benjamin, A. E. (1989). Chronic care: Perspectives on AIDS and aging. *Generations, 13*(4), 19-22.

Benjamin, M., & Curtis, J. (1992). *Ethics in nursing* (3rd ed.). New York: Oxford University Press.

Bennett, C. L., Pascal, A., & Cvitanic, M. (1992). Medical care costs of intravenous drug users with AIDS in Brooklyn. *Journal of Acquired Immune Deficiency Syndrome, 5*(1), 1-6.

Bennett, M. J. (1990). Stigmatization: Experiences of persons with acquired immune deficiency syndrome. *Issues in Mental Health Nursing, 11,* 141-154.

Beresford, L. (1989). Alternative, outpatient settings of care for people with AIDS. *Quarterly Review Bulletin, 15,* 9-16.

Bilheimer, L. T., Asher, A., Phillips, B., & Smith, M. (1991). A modeling framework for AIDS/HIV nonacute care services. *Quarterly Review Bulletin, 17,* 216-228.

Bishop, A. H., & Scudder, J. R., Jr. (1990). *The practical, moral, and personal sense of nursing.* Albany: SUNY Press.

Blanchet, K. D. (1990). Effective HIV testing strategies for chemical dependency programs. *AIDS Patient Care, 4,* 21-23.

Blendon, R. J., & Donelan, K. (1990). AIDS and discrimination: Public and professional perspectives. In L. O. Gostin (Ed.), *AIDS and the health care system* (pp. 77-84). New Haven, CT: Yale University Press.

Blendon, R. J., Donelan, K., & Knox, R. A. (1992). Public opinion and AIDS: Lessons for the second decade. *Journal of the American Medical Association, 267,* 981-986.

Bloom, D. E., & Glied, S. (1991). Benefits and costs of HIV testing. *Science, 252,* 1798-1804.

Blum, L. A. (1988). Gilligan and Kohlberg: Implications for moral theory. *Ethics, 98,* 472-491.

Boekeloo, B. O., Marx, E. S., Kral, A. H., Coughlin, S. C., Bowman, M., & Rabin, D. L. (1991). Frequency and thoroughness of STD/HIV risk assessment by physicians in a high-risk metropolitan area. *American Journal of Public Health, 81,* 1645-1648.

Boland, M. G., & Conviser, R. (1992). Nursing care of the child. In J. H. Flaskerud & P. J. Ungvarski (Eds.), *HIV/AIDS: A guide to nursing care* (pp. 199-238). Philadelphia: W. B. Saunders.

Boyd, K. M. (1990). HIV infection: The ethics of anonymised testing and of testing pregnant women. *Journal of Medical Ethics, 16,* 173-178.

Boyle, L. R., & Senay, E. C. (1991). HIV prevention education for intravenous drug users awaiting admission to drug treatment. *AIDS Patient Care, 5,* 301-303.

Brennan, T. A. (1989). Removing barriers to health care for people with HIV-related disease: A matter of law or ethics. In D. E. Rogers & E. Ginzberg (Eds.), *Public and professional attitudes toward AIDS patients* (pp. 55-73). San Francisco: Westview.

Brennan, T. A. (1991). Transmission of the human immunodeficiency virus in the health care setting. *The New England Journal of Medicine, 324,* 1504-1509.

Brock, D. W. (1991). The ideal of shared decision making between physicians and patients. *Kennedy Institute of Ethics Journal, 1,* 28-47.

Brock, D. W. (1992). Voluntary active euthanasia. *Hastings Center Report, 22*(2), 10-22.

Brooks-Gunn, J., & Furstenberg, F. F., Jr. (1990). Coming of age in the era of AIDS. *The Milbank Quarterly, 68,* 59-84.

Brown, M. A., & Powell-Cope, G. M. (1991). AIDS family caregiving: Transitions through uncertainty. *Nursing Research, 40,* 338-345.

Brown, Y., Calder, B., & Rae, D. (1990). The effect of knowledge on nursing students' attitudes toward individuals with AIDS. *Journal of Nursing Education, 29,* 367-372.

Buck, B. A. (1991). Support groups for hospitalized AIDS patients. *AIDS Patient Care, 5,* 255-258.

Cady, J., & Hunter, K. M. (1989). Making contact: The AIDS plays. In E. T. Juengst & B. A. Koenig (Eds.), *The meaning of AIDS: Implications for medical science, clinical practice, and public health policy* (pp. 42-49). New York: Praeger.

Callahan, D. (1990). Religion and the secularization of bioethics. *Hastings Center Report, 20*(4), 2-4.

Calsyn, D. A., Saxon, A. J., Freeman, G., Jr., & Whittaker, S. (1992). Ineffectiveness of AIDS education and HIV antibody testing in reducing high-risk behaviors among injection drug users. *American Journal of Public Health, 82,* 573-575.

Cameron, M. (1986). The moral and ethical component of nurse burnout. *Nursing Management, 17*(4), 42B-42E.

Cameron, M. E. (1991a). Ethical problems experienced by persons with AIDS (Doctoral dissertation, University of Minnesota, 1991). *Dissertation Abstracts International, 52/06B,* 2990.

Cameron, M. (1991b). Virtue, justice and caring. *Journal of Professional Nursing, 7*, 206.

Cameron, M. E., & Schaffer, M. A. (1992). Tell me the right answer: A model for teaching nursing ethics. *Journal of Nursing Education, 31*, 377-380.

Campbell, C. S. (1990). Religion and moral meaning in bioethics. *Hastings Center Report, 20*(4), 4-10.

Campbell, C. S. (1991). Ethics and militant AIDS activism. In F. G. Reamer (Ed.), *AIDS & ethics* (pp. 155-187). New York: Columbia University Press.

Campbell, S., Maki, M., Willenbring, K., & Henry, K. (1991). AIDS-related knowledge, attitudes, and behaviors among 629 registered nurses at a Minnesota hospital: A descriptive study. *Journal of Nurses in AIDS Care, 2*(1), 15-23.

Capell, F. J., Vugia, D. J., Mordaunt, V. L., Marelich, W. D., Ascher, M. S., Trachtenberg, A. I., Cunningham, G. C., Arnon, S. S., & Kizer, K. W. (1992). Distribution of HIV Type 1 Infection in childbearing women in California. *American Journal of Public Health, 82*, 254-256.

Carmack, B. J. (1992). Balancing engagement/detachment in AIDS-related multiple losses. *Image: Journal of Nursing Scholarship, 24*, 9-14.

Carrick, P. (1989). AIDS: Ethical, legal, and public policy implications. In E. T. Juengst & B. A. Koenig (Eds.), *The meaning of AIDS: Implications for medical science, clinical practice, and public health policy* (pp. 163-173). New York: Praeger.

Cassidy, C. E. (1991). Surveying home health care workers regarding AIDS. *AIDS Patient Care, 5*, 304-311.

Centers for Disease Control. (1987). Revision of the CDC surveillance case definition for acquired immunodeficiency syndrome. *Morbidity and Mortality Weekly Report, 36* (Suppl. 1S), 1S-15S.

Centers for Disease Control. (1991a, April). *HIV/AIDS surveillance report.* Atlanta: Division of HIV/AIDS.

Centers for Disease Control. (1991b). Review of draft for revision of HIV infection classification system and expansion of AIDS surveillance case definition. *Morbidity and Mortality Weekly Report, 40*, 787.

Centers for Disease Control. (1992a, March). *HIV/AIDS surveillance report.* Atlanta: Division of HIV/AIDS.

Centers for Disease Control. (1992b). Selected behaviors that increase risk for HIV infection among high school students—United States, 1990. *Morbidity and Mortality Weekly Report, 41*, 231-240.

Chang, S. W., Katz, M. H., & Hernandez, S. R. (1992). The new AIDS case definition. *Journal of the American Medical Association, 267*, 973-975.

Childress, J. F. (1991). Mandatory HIV screening and testing. In F. G. Reamer (Ed.), *AIDS & ethics* (pp. 50-76). New York: Columbia University Press.

Chitwood, D. D., Inciardi, J. A., McBride, D. C., McCoy, C. B., McCoy, H. V., & Trapido, E. (1991). *A community approach to AIDS intervention.* Westport, CT: Greenwood Press.

Cleary, P. D., Van Devanter, N., Rogers, T. F., Singer, E., Shipton-Levy, R., Steilen, M., Stuart, A., Avorn, J., & Pindyck, J. (1991). Behavior change after notification of HIV infection. *American Journal of Public Health, 81*, 1586-1590.

Cline, R. J. W., Johnson, S. J., & Freeman, K. E. (1992). Talk among sexual partners about AIDS: Interpersonal communication for risk reduction or risk enhancement? *Health Communication, 4*(1), 39-56.

Cockerell, C. J., & Nary, G. (1991). AIDS, discrimination, and access to health care. *AIDS Patient Care, 5,* 2-3.

Cohen, F. L. (1991). The clinical spectrum of HIV infection and its treatment. In J. D. Durham & F. L. Cohen (Eds.), *The person with AIDS* (2nd ed.) (pp. 135-205). New York: Springer.

Colby, D. C., & Cook, T. E. (1991). Epidemics and agendas: The politics of nightly news coverage of AIDS. *Journal of Health Politics, Policy and Law, 16,* 215-249.

Coles, R. (1989). *The call of stories.* Boston: Houghton Mifflin.

Condon, E. H. (1992). Nursing and the caring metaphor: Gender and political influences on an ethics of care. *Nursing Outlook, 40,* 14-19.

Cooper, M. C. (1990). Reconceptualizing nursing ethics. *Scholarly Inquiry for Nursing Practice, 4,* 209-218.

Cooper, M. C. (1991). Principle-oriented ethics and the ethic of care: A creative tension. *Advances in Nursing Science, 14*(2), 22-31.

Cooper, T., & Weiss, R. (1989). HIV infection and AIDS: Recommendations to the President-Elect. In D. E. Rogers & E. Ginzberg (Eds.), *Public and professional attitudes toward AIDS patients* (pp. 97-110). San Francisco: Westview.

Coulter, A. (1991). Speaking out against mandatory HIV testing for health care workers. *AIDS Patient Care, 5,* 110-115.

Crimp, D. (Ed.). (1988). *AIDS: Cultural analysis/cultural activism.* Cambridge: MIT Press.

Crisham, C. (1985). Resolving ethical and moral dilemmas of nursing interventions. In M. Snyder (Ed.), *Independent nursing interventions* (pp. 25-43). New York: John Wiley.

Dahl, N. (1987). Morality and the meaning of life. *Canadian Journal of Philosophy, 17*(1), 1-22.

Daniels, N. (1990). Insurability and the HIV epidemic. *The Milbank Quarterly, 68,* 497-525.

Daniels, N. (1991). Duty to treat or right to refuse? *Hastings Center Report, 21*(2), 36-46.

Daniels, N. (1992). HIV-infected health care professionals: Public threat or public sacrifice? *The Milbank Quarterly, 70,* 3-42.

Danila, R. N., MacDonald, K. L., Rhame, F. S., Moen, M. E., Reier, D. O., LeTourneau, J. C., Sheehan, M. K., Armstrong, J., Bender, M. E., Osterholm, M. T., & the Investigation Team. (1991). A look-back investigation of patients of an HIV-infected physician. *The New England Journal of Medicine, 325,* 1406-1411.

Danis, M., & Churchill, L. R. (1991). Autonomy and the common weal. *Hastings Center Report, 21*(1), 25-31.

Davis, A. J. (1989). Ethical issues in nursing research. *Western Journal of Nursing Research, 11,* 632.

Davis, A. J. (1991). The allocation of health care resources. *Western Journal of Nursing Research, 13,* 136-137.

Decker, J. F. (1987). Prostitution as a public health issue. In H. L. Dalton, S. Burris, & the Yale AIDS Law Project (Eds.), *AIDS and the law: A guide for the public* (pp. 81-89). New Haven, CT: Yale University Press.

Department of Labor. (1989, May 30). *Federal Register, Part II, 54,* 23042-23139.

DePhilippis, D., Metzger, D. S., Woody, G. E., & Navaline, H. A. (1992). Attitudes toward mandatory human immunodeficiency virus testing and contact tracing. *Journal of Substance Abuse Treatment, 9,* 39-42.

Doll, L. S., Petersen, L. R., White, C. R., Johnson, E. S., Ward, J. W., & the Blood Donor Study Group. (1992). Homosexually and nonhomosexually identified men who have sex with men: A behavioral comparison. *The Journal of Sex Research, 29,* 1-14.

Downes, J. (1991). Acquired immunodeficiency syndrome: The nurse's legal duty to serve. *Journal of Professional Nursing, 7,* 333-340.

Dresser, R. (1992). Wanted: Single, white male for medical research. *Hastings Center Report, 22*(1), 24-29.

Driedger, S. M., & Cox, D. (1991). Burnout in nurses who care for PWAs. *AIDS Patient Care, 5,* 197-203.

Durham, J. E. (1991). The HIV epidemic: Ethical and legal dimensions. In J. D. Durham & F. L. Cohen (Eds.), *The person with AIDS* (2nd ed.) (pp. 361-387). New York: Springer.

Eakes, G. G. (1990). Grief resolution in hospice nurses. *Nursing & Health Care, 11,* 243-248.

Earickson, R. J. (1990). International behavioral responses to a health hazard: AIDS. *Social Science and Medicine, 31,* 951-962.

Edgar, H., & Rothman, D. J. (1990). New rules for new drugs. *The Milbank Quarterly, 68,* 111-142.

Efantis, J. (1991). The impact of HIV infection on women. In J. D. Durham & F. L. Cohen (Eds.), *The person with AIDS: Nursing perspectives* (2nd ed.) (pp. 300-315). New York: Springer.

Eliason, M. J., & Randall, C. E. (1991). Lesbian phobia in nursing students. *Western Journal of Nursing Research, 13,* 363-374.

El-Sadr, W., & Capps, L. (1992). The challenge of minority recruitment in clinical trials for AIDS. *Journal of the American Medical Association, 267,* 954-957.

Faber-Langendoen, K., & Bartels, D. M. (1992). Process of forgoing life-sustaining treatment in a university hospital: An empirical study. *Critical Care Medicine, 20,* 570-577.

Faden, R. R., Geller, G., & Powers, M. (1991). *AIDS, women, and the next generation.* New York: Oxford University Press.

Fahs, M. C., Fulop, G., Strain, J., Sacks, H. S., Muller, C., Cleary, P. D., Schmeidler, J., & Turner, B. (1992). The inpatient AIDS unit: A preliminary empirical investigation of access, economic, and outcome issues. *American Journal of Public Health, 82,* 576-578.

Ficarrotto, J. J., Grade, M., & Zegans, L. S. (1991). Occupational and personal risk estimates for HIV contagion among incoming graduate nursing students. *Journal of the Association of Nurses in AIDS Care, 2*(1), 5-11.

Fielstein, E. M., Fielstein, L. L., & Hazelwood, M. G. (1992). AIDS knowledge among college freshmen students: Need for education? *Journal of Sex Education and Therapy, 18,* 45-54.

Fins, J. J. (1992). Palliation in the age of chronic disease. *Hastings Center Report, 22*(1), 41-42.

Flack, H. E., & Pellegrino, E. D. (Eds.). (1992). *African-American perspectives on biomedical ethics.* Washington, DC: Georgetown University Press.

Flanagan, N. (1990). DNR and AIDS: Who decides? *AIDS Patient Care, 4,* 38-41.

Flanagan, O., & Jackson, I. (1987). Justice, care, and gender. *Ethics, 97,* 622-637.

Flaskerud, J. H. (1992). Psychosocial aspects. In J. H. Flaskerud & P. J. Ungvarski (Eds.), *HIV/AIDS: A guide to nursing care* (pp. 239-274). Philadelphia: W. B. Saunders.

Flaskerud, J. H., & Ungvarski, P. J. (1992). *HIV/AIDS: A guide to nursing care* (2nd ed.). Philadelphia: W. B. Saunders.

Fleck, L. (1991). Please don't tell! *Hastings Center Report, 21*(6), 39-40.

Forrester, D. A. (1990). AIDS-related risk factors, medical diagnosis, do-not-resuscitate orders and aggressiveness of nursing care. *Nursing Research, 39*, 350-354.

Fortunato, J. E. (1987). *AIDS: The spiritual dilemma*. San Francisco: Harper & Row.

Fowler, M. D. M. (1988a). Acquired immunodeficiency syndrome and refusal to provide care. *Heart & Lung, 17*, 213-215.

Fowler, M. D. M. (1988b). Issues in qualitative research. *Western Journal of Nursing Research, 10*, 109-111.

Fox, D. M. (1987). Physicians versus lawyers: A conflict of cultures. In H. L. Dalton, S. Burris, & the Yale AIDS Law Project (Eds.), *AIDS and the law: A guide for the public* (pp. 210-217). New Haven, CT: Yale University Press.

Fox, D. M. (1990). Chronic disease and disadvantage. *Journal of Health Politics, Policy and Law, 15*, 341-355.

Fox, D. M., & Thomas, E. H. (1990). The cost of AIDS: Exaggeration, entitlement, and economics. In L. O. Gostin (Ed.), *AIDS and the health care system* (pp. 197-210). New Haven, CT: Yale University Press.

Fox, R. C., Aiken, L. H., & Messikomer, C. M. (1990). The culture of caring: AIDS and the nursing profession. *The Milbank Quarterly, 68*, 226-256.

Frankena, W. K. (1973). *Ethics* (2nd ed.). Englewood Cliffs, NJ: Prentice-Hall.

Freedman, B., & McGill/Boston Research Group. (1989). Nonvalidated therapies and HIV disease. *Hastings Center Report, 19*(3), 14-20.

Freeman, E. (1992). Difficult choices. *Journal of Nurses in AIDS Care, 3*(1), 5.

Friedman, S. R., DesJarlais, D. C., & Sterk, C. E. (1990). AIDS and the social relations of intravenous drug users. *The Milbank Quarterly, 68*, 85-110.

Fry, S. T. (1989). Toward a theory of nursing ethics. *Advances in Nursing Science, 11*(4), 9-22.

Fuerst, M. L. (1991). Cost analysis of AIDS outpatient services. *AIDS Patient Care, 5*, 31-33.

Funkhouser, S. W., & Moser, D. K. (1990). Is health care racist? *Advances in Nursing Science, 12*(2), 47-55.

Gallop, R. M., Lancee, W. J., Taerk, G., Coates, R. A., & Fanning, M. (1992). Fear of contagion and AIDS: Nurses' perception of risk. *AIDS Care, 4*, 103-109.

Gaskins, S., Sowell, R., & Gueldner, S. (1991). Overcoming methodological barriers to HIV/AIDS nursing research. *Journal of Association of Nurses in AIDS Care, 2*, 33-37.

Gee, G. (1989). Nurse attitudes and AIDS. In D. E. Rogers & E. Ginzberg (Eds.), *Public and professional attitudes toward AIDS patients* (pp. 43-53). San Francisco: Westview.

Gemson, D. H., Colombotos, J., Elinson, J., Fordyce, E. J., Hynes, M., & Stoneburner, R. (1991). Acquired immunodeficiency syndrome prevention. *Archives of Internal Medicine, 151*, 1102-1108.

Gilligan, C. (1982). *In a different voice: Psychological theory and women's development*. Cambridge, MA: Harvard University Press.

Glantz, L. H., Mariner, W. K., & Annas, G. J. (1992). Risky business: Setting public health policy for HIV-infected health care professionals. *The Milbank Quarterly, 70*, 43-79.

Glover, J. J., & Starkeson, E. C. (1989). Health care professionals and the potential for iatrogenic transmission of AIDS. In E. T. Juengst & B. A. Koenig (Eds.), *The meaning of AIDS: Implications for medical science, clinical practice, and public health policy* (pp. 152-162). New York: Praeger.

Gold, J. A., Jablonski, D. F., Christensen, P. J., Shapiro, R. S., & Schiedermayer, D. L. (1990). Is there a right to futile treatment? The case of a dying patient with AIDS. *The Journal of Clinical Ethics, 1*, 19-23.

Goldman, D. S., & Stryker, J. (1991). The national commission on AIDS. *Kennedy Institute of Ethics Journal, 1*, 339-345.

Goldstein, R. (1990). The implicated and the immune. *The Milbank Quarterly, 68*, 295-320.

Gostin, L. (1987). Traditional public health strategies. In H. L. Dalton, S. Burris, & the Yale AIDS Law Project (Eds.), *AIDS and the law: A guide for the public* (pp. 47-65). New Haven, CT: Yale University Press.

Grady, C. (1992). Ethical Aspects. In J. H. Flaskerud & P. J. Ungvarski (Eds.), *HIV/AIDS: A guide to nursing care* (pp. 424-439). Philadelphia: W. B. Saunders.

Green, R. (1987). The transmission of AIDS. In H. L. Dalton, S. Burris, & the Yale AIDS Law Project (Eds.), *AIDS and the law: A guide for the public* (pp. 28-36). New Haven, CT: Yale University Press.

Grossman, A. H. (1991). Gay men and HIV/AIDS: Understanding the double stigma. *Journal of Nurses in AIDS Care, 2*(4), 28-32.

Grund, J.-P. C., Kaplan, C. D., & Adriaans, N. F. P. (1991). Needle sharing in the Netherlands: An ethnographic analysis. *American Journal of Public Health, 81*, 1602-1607.

Gwartney, D. L., Daly, P. B., Roccaforte, J. S., & Smith, P. W. (1992). PWAs in the long term care facility. *AIDS Patient Care, 6*, 15-18.

Gwin, M. (1991). Prevalence of HIV infection in childbearing women in the United States. *Journal of the American Medical Association, 265*, 1704-1708.

Hall, J. M., & Stevens, P. E. (1991). Rigor in feminist research. *Advances in Nursing Science, 13*(3), 16-29.

Hallie, P. (1989). From cruelty to goodness. In C. Sommers & F. Sommers (Eds.), *Vice and virtue in everyday life* (pp. 9-24), New York: Harcourt Brace Jovanovich.

Hartgers, C., van den Hoek, A., Krijnen, P., & Coutinho, R. A. (1992). HIV prevalence and risk behavior among injecting drug users who participate in "low-threshold" methadone programs in Amsterdam. *American Journal of Public Health, 82*, 547-551.

Heagarty, M. C., & Abrams, E. J. (1992). Caring for HIV-infected women and children. *The New England Journal of Medicine, 326*, 887-888.

Hinman, A. R. (1991). Strategies to prevent HIV infection in the United States. *American Journal of Public Health, 81*, 1557-1559.

Hitchcock, J. M., & Wilson, H. S. (1992). Personal risking: Lesbian self-disclosure of sexual orientation to professional health care providers. *Nursing Research, 41*, 178-183.

Hoagland, S. L. (1990). Some concerns about Nel Noddings' *Caring. Hypatia, 5*(1), 109-114.

Houston, B. (1990). Caring and exploitation. *Hypatia, 5*(1), 115-119.

Husted, G. L., & Husted, J. H. (1991). *Ethical decision making in nursing*. St. Louis: C. V. Mosby.

Hutchison, M., & Kurth, A. (1991). "I need to know that I have a choice." *AIDS Patient Care, 5,* 17-25.

Hutman, S. (1991). Choosing the best hospital for AIDS care. *AIDS Patient Care, 5,* 6-8.

Jecker, N. S. (1990). The responsibility to treat AIDS patients. *AIDS Patient Care, 4,* 2-4.

Jemmott, L. S., & Jemmott, J. B., III. (1991). Applying the theory of reasoned action to AIDS risk behavior: Condom use among black women. *Nursing Research, 40,* 228-234.

Jemmott, L. S., Jemmott, J. B., III, & Cruz-Collins, M. (1992). Predicting AIDS patient care intentions among nursing students. *Nursing Research, 41,* 172-177.

Jennings, B., Callahan, D., & Caplan, A. L. (1988). Ethical challenges of chronic illness. *Hastings Center Report, 18*(1), 1-16.

Jonas, H. (1992). The burden and blessing of mortality. *Hastings Center Report, 22*(1), 34-40.

Kant, I. (1986). *Grounding for the metaphysics of morals* (J. W. Ellington, Trans.). Indianapolis, IN: Hackett Publishing.

Karpen, M. (1990). A comprehensive world overview of needle exchange programs. *AIDS Patient Care, 4*(4), 26-28.

Kass, N. E., Faden, R. R., Fox, R., & Dudley, J. (1991). Loss of private health insurance among homosexual men with AIDS. *Inquiry, 28,* 249-254.

Kendall, J. (1992). Promoting wellness in HIV-support groups. *Journal of the Association of Nurses in AIDS Care, 3*(1), 28-38.

King, P. A. (1991). Helping women helping children: Drug policy and future generations. *The Milbank Quarterly, 69,* 595-622.

Knox, M. D., & Gaies, J. S. (1992). The HIV clinical tutorial for community mental health professionals. *AIDS Patient Care, 6,* 34-37.

Kobasa, S.C.O. (1990). AIDS and volunteer associations. *The Milbank Quarterly, 68,* 280-294.

Kohlberg, L. (1983). *The psychology of moral development* (Vol. 2). New York: Harper & Row.

Larson, E., & Ropka, M. E. (1991). An update on nursing research and HIV infection. *Image: Journal of Nursing Scholarship, 23,* 4-12.

Levin, B. W., Driscoll, J. M., & Fleischman, A. R. (1991). Treatment choice for infants in the neonatal intensive care unit at risk for AIDS. *Journal of the American Medical Association, 265,* 2976-2981.

Levine, C. (1990a). AIDS and changing concepts of family. *The Milbank Quarterly, 68,* 33-58.

Levine, C. (1990b). In and out of the hospital. In L. O. Gostin (Ed.), *AIDS and the health care system* (pp. 45-61). New Haven, CT: Yale University Press.

Levine, C. (1991). AIDS and the ethics of human subjects research. In F. G. Reamer (Ed.), *AIDS & ethics* (pp. 77-104). New York: Columbia University Press.

Levine, R. J. (1991). AIDS and the physician-patient relationship. In F. G. Reamer (Ed.), *AIDS & ethics* (pp. 188-214). New York: Columbia University Press.

Levinson, G., & Miller, R. L. (1992). HIV-related walk-in peer counseling. *AIDS Patient Care, 6,* 28-33.

Lewis, C. E., & Coffee, J. (1991). Public health nurses and AIDS. *Nursing Outlook, 39*, 132-135.

Lewis, J. B., & Eakes, G. G. (1992). The AIDS care dilemma: An exercise in critical thinking. *Journal of Nursing Education, 31*, 136-137.

Lewis, L. (1989). AIDS as a chronic disease. *AIDS Patient Care, 3*, 28-30.

Lo, B. (1989). Life-sustaining treatment in patients with AIDS. In E. T. Juengst & B. A. Koenig (Eds.), *The meaning of AIDS: Implications for medical science, clinical practice, and public health policy* (pp. 86-93). New York: Praeger.

Lo, B., & Steinbrook, R. (1992). Health care workers infected with the human immunodeficiency virus. *Journal of the American Medical Association, 267*, 1100-1105.

Loewy, E. H. (1992). Healing and killing, harming and not harming: Physician participation in euthanasia and capital punishment. *The Journal of Clinical Ethics, 3*, 29-34.

Lombardo, J. M., Kloser, P. C., Pawel, B. R., Trost, R. C., Kapila, R., & St. Louis, M. E. (1991). Anonymous human immunodeficiency virus surveillance and clinical directed testing in a Newark, NJ, hospital. *Archives of Internal Medicine, 151*, 965-968.

Lovejoy, N. C. (1991). Arguments against mandatory screening for HIV in low-prevalence areas. *Journal of Association of Nurses in AIDS Care, 2*(2), 7-14.

Lynch, C. A. (1992). The revised CDC case definition. *Journal of the Association of Nurses in AIDS Care, 3*(1), 45-47.

Macklin, R. (1991). HIV-infected psychiatric patients: Beyond confidentiality. *Ethics and Behavior, 1*, 3-20.

Mandelker, D. R. (1987). Housing issues. In H. L. Dalton, S. Burris, & the Yale AIDS Law Project (Eds.), *AIDS and the law: A guide for the public* (pp. 142-152). New Haven, CT: Yale University Press.

Manzella, J. P., Falk, S. Y., McConville, J. H., & Kellogg, J. A. (1992). Impact of the counselor on rates of informed consent and pre and posttest HIV counseling. *AIDS Patient Care, 6*, 19-20.

Marks, G., Richardson, J. L., & Maldonado, N. (1991). Self-disclosure of HIV infection to sexual partners. *American Journal of Public Health, 81*, 1321-1323.

Martin, D. A. (1990). Effects of ethical dilemmas on stress felt by nurses providing care to AIDS patients. *Critical Care Nursing Quarterly, 12*(4), 53-62.

Matens, R. W. (1991). Cultural sensitivity in AIDS education for the Hispanic community. *AIDS Patient Care, 5*, 140-142.

Mattingly, S. S. (1992). The maternal-fetal dyad. *Hastings Center Report, 22*(1), 13-18.

May, W. F. (1992). The beleaguered rulers: The public obligation of the professional. *Kennedy Institute of Ethics Journal, 2*(1), 25-41.

McCaig, L. F., Hardy, A. M., & Winn, D. M. (1991). The US adult population: Influence of the local incidence of AIDS. *American Journal of Public Health, 81*, 1591-1595.

McCusker, J., Stoddard, A. M., & McCarthy, E. (1992). The validity of self-reported HIV antibody test results. *American Journal of Public Health, 82*, 567-569.

McCusker, J., Stoddard, A. M., Zapka, J. G., Morrison, C. S., Zorn, M., & Lewis, B. F. (1992). AIDS education for drug abusers: Evaluation of short-term effectiveness. *American Journal of Public Health, 82*, 533-540.

McNabb, K., & Keller, M. L. (1991). Nurses' risk taking regarding HIV transmission in the workplace. *Western Journal of Nursing Research, 13,* 732-745.

Meier, D. E. (1992). Physician-assisted dying: Theory and reality. *The Journal of Clinical Ethics, 3*(1), 35-37.

Meisenhelder, J. B. (1991). Fear of contagion among home health aides: A community survey. *Journal of Association of Nurses in AIDS Care, 2*(1), 31-35.

Moore, P. A. (1991). Treating HIV infection as a chronic disease. *AIDS Patient Care, 5,* 113-139.

Moritz, P. (1990). *Bioethics and clinical practice.* Washington, DC: National Center for Nursing Research.

Moseley, R. E. (1989). AIDS and the allocation of intensive care unit beds. In E. T. Juengst & B. A. Koenig (Eds.), *The meaning of AIDS: Implications for medical science, clinical practice, and public health policy* (pp. 101-107). New York: Praeger.

Murphy, T. F. (1988). Is AIDS a just punishment? *Journal of Medical Ethics, 14,* 154-160.

Murphy, T. F. (1990). Reproductive controls and sexual destiny. *Bioethics, 4,* 121-142.

Murphy, T. F. (1991a). The ethics of conversion therapy. *Bioethics, 5,* 123-138.

Murphy, T. F. (1991b). No time for an AIDS backlash. *Hastings Center Report, 21*(2), 7-11.

Murphy, T. F. (1991c). The politics of AIDS. *Medical Humanities Review, 5,* 87-92.

Murphy, T. F. (1991d). Women and drug users: The changing faces of HIV clinical drug trials. *Quarterly Review Bulletin, 17,* 26-32.

Murphy, T. F. (1992). Legal liability for pregnant women with HIV? *Medical Ethics, 7,* 3-4.

Murphy, T. F., & Poirier, S. (1993). *Writing AIDS: Gay literature, language, and analysis.* New York: Columbia University Press.

National Center for Nursing Research. (1990). *HIV infection: Prevention and care.* Bethesda, MD: U.S. Department of Health and Human Services.

National League for Nursing. (1988). *AIDS guidelines for schools of nursing.* New York: Author.

Nelkin, D. (1991). AIDS and the news media. *The Milbank Quarterly, 69,* 293-307.

Nelkin, D., Willis, D. P., & Parris, S. V. (1990). Introduction. *The Milbank Quarterly, 68,* 1-9.

Nelson, H. L. (1991). AIDS & entrepreneurs. *Hastings Center Report, 21*(6), 2-3.

New York Academy of Medicine. (1991). The risk of contracting HIV infection in the course of health care. *Journal of the American Medical Association, 265,* 1872-1873.

Noddings, N. (1984). *Caring: A feminine approach to ethics and moral education.* Los Angeles: University of California Press.

Noddings, N. (1990). Review symposium. *Hypatia, 5*(1), 120-126.

Nokes, K. M. (1992). HIV infection in women. In J. H. Flaskerud & P. J. Ungvarski (Eds.), *HIV/AIDS: A guide to nursing care* (pp. 375-396). Philadelphia: W. B. Saunders.

Nokes, K. M., & Carver, K. (1991). The meaning of living with AIDS. *Nursing Science Quarterly, 4,* 175-179.

Nouwen, H. J. M. (1979). *The wounded healer.* Garden City, NY: Doubleday.

Obermeyer, T. E., & Streeter, A. (1991). Street outreach HIV education to intravenous drug users and other substance users. *AIDS Patient Care, 5,* 312-314.

Oiler, C. J. (1986). Phenomenology. In P. L. Munhall & C. J. Oiler (Eds.), *Nursing research* (pp. 69-83). Norwalk, CT: Appleton-Century-Crofts.

O'Neil, M. (1989). Grief and bereavement in AIDS and aging. *Generations, 13*(4), 80-82.

O'Neill, C. (1987). Intravenous drug abusers. In H. L. Dalton, S. Burris, & the Yale AIDS Law Project (Eds.), *AIDS and the law: A guide for the public* (pp. 253-280). New Haven, CT: Yale University Press.

Oppenheimer, G. M., & Padgug, R. A. (1991). AIDS and the crisis of health insurance. In F. G. Reamer (Ed.), *AIDS & ethics* (pp. 105-127). New York: Columbia University Press.

Parker, R. S. (1990). Measuring nurses' moral judgments. *Image: Journal of Nursing Scholarship, 22*, 213-218.

Pellegrino, E., & Thomasma, D. C. (1988). *For the patient's good: The restoration of beneficence in health care.* New York: Oxford University Press.

Pfeiffer, N. (1992). Long-term survival and HIV disease. *AIDS Patient Care, 6*, 134-137.

Phillips, J. R. (1992). Choosing and participating in the living-dying process: A research emergent. *Nursing Science Quarterly, 5*, 4-5.

Pierce, C., & VanDeVeer, D. (1988). *AIDS: Ethics and public policy.* Belmont, CA: Wadsworth.

Plato. (1961). *Symposium* (W.R.M. Lamb, Trans.). Cambridge, MA: Harvard University Press.

Poku, K. A. (1992). Knowingly exposing others to HIV. *AIDS Patient Care, 6*, 5-10.

Powers, M. (1990). Ethical considerations in HIV screening programs for infected women and children. *AIDS Patient Care, 4*, 40-41.

Priester, R. (1992). A values framework for health system reform. *Health Affairs, 11*, 84-107.

Primm, B. (1990). Needle exchange programs do not solve the problems of HIV transmission. *AIDS Patient Care, 4*, 18-20.

Purdon, J. E. (1992). Fear of persons with HIV infection: Teaching strategies for helping students cope. *Journal of Nursing Education, 31*, 138-139.

Quill, T. E. (1991). Bad news: Delivery, dialogue, and dilemmas. *Archives of Internal Medicine, 151*, 463-468.

Ragsdale, D., Kotarba, J. A., & Morrow, J. R. (1992). Work-related activities to improve quality of life in HIV disease. *Journal of Nurses in AIDS Care, 3*(1), 39-44.

Ragsdale, D., & Morrow, J. R. (1990). Quality of life as a function of HIV classification. *Nursing Research, 39*, 355-358.

Ramos, M. C. (1989). Some ethical implications of qualitative research. *Research in Nursing & Health, 12*, 57-63.

Raveis, V. H., & Siegel, K. (1991). The impact of care giving on informal or familial care givers. *AIDS Patient Care, 5*, 39-43.

Raviglione, M. C., Battan, R., Garner, G., Cortes, H., Sugar, J., & Taranta, A. (1992). Risk of exposure to HIV-infected body fluids among medical housestaff. *AIDS Patient Care, 6*, 52-55.

Reamer, F. G. (Ed.). (1991). *AIDS & ethics.* New York: Columbia University Press.

Rest, J. R. (1986). *Moral development: Advances in research and theory.* New York: Praeger.

Rogers, B. (1989). AIDS and ethics in the workplace. *Nursing Outlook, 37*(6), 254, 255, 290.

Rogers, D. E. (1989). Summation: Better care of AIDS patients. In D. E. Rogers & E. Ginzberg (Eds.), *Public and professional attitudes toward AIDS patients* (pp. 119-124). San Francisco: Westview.

Rothman, D. J., & Tynan, E. A. (1990). Advantages and disadvantages of special hospitals for patients with HIV infection. *The New England Journal of Medicine, 323,* 764-768.

Rousseau, J. J. (1979). *Emile: Or on education* (A. Bloom, Trans.). New York: Basic Books.

St. Onge, J. L. (1992). Codependence: Addictive relationships and HIV care. *AIDS Patient Care, 6,* 25-27.

Sandelowski, M. (1991). Telling stories: Narrative approaches in qualitative research. *Image: Journal of Nursing Scholarship, 23,* 161-166.

Schoeman, F. (1991). AIDS and privacy. In F. G. Reamer (Ed.), *AIDS & ethics* (pp. 240-276). New York: Columbia University Press.

Schulman, D. I. (1992). Stigma, risk, and the Florida AIDS dental cases. *AIDS Patient Care, 6,* 3-4.

Schulman, K. A., Lynn, L. A., Glick, H. A., & Eisenberg, J. M. (1991). Cost effectiveness of low-dose zidovudine therapy for asymptomatic patients with human immunodeficiency virus (HIV) infection. *Annals of Internal Medicine, 114,* 798-802.

Schwarz, J. K. (1992). Living wills and health care proxies: Nursing practice implications. *Nursing & Health Care, 13,* 92-96.

Schwarz, M. R. (1989). Physicians' attitudes toward AIDS. In D. E. Rogers & E. Ginzberg (Eds.), *Public and professional attitudes toward AIDS patients* (pp. 31-41). San Francisco: Westview.

Shilts, R. (1987). *And the band played on.* New York: St. Martin's.

Siegal, H. A., Carlson, R. G., Falck, R., Li, L., Forney, M. A., Rapp, R. C., Baumgartner, K., Myers, W., & Nelson, M. (1991). HIV infection and risk behavior among intravenous drug users in low seroprevalence areas in the Midwest. *American Journal of Public Health, 81,* 1642-1644.

Silverman, D., Perakyla, A., & Bor, R. (1992). Discussing safer sex in HIV counselling: Assessing three communication formats. *AIDS Care, 4,* 69-82.

Smart, J.J.S., & Williams, B. (1985). *Utilitarianism: For and against.* New York: Cambridge University Press.

Smeltzer, S. C., & Whipple, B. (1991). Women and HIV infection. *Image: Journal of Nursing Scholarship, 23,* 249-256.

Smith, J. E., Stevenson, L. Y., Keeling, R., & Herrick, C. A. (1989). Everyday ethics in AIDS care. *AIDS Patient Care, 3,* 27-31.

Smith, J. R., Forster, G. E., Kitchen, V. S., Hool, Y. S., Munday, P. E., & Paintin, D. B. (1991). Infertility management in HIV positive couples: A dilemma. *British Medical Journal, 302,* 1447-1450.

Sommers, C., & Sommers, F. (1989). *Vice & virtue in everyday life.* New York: Harcourt Brace Jovanovich.

Sontag, S. (1989). *AIDS and its metaphors.* New York: Farrar, Straus & Giroux.

Sorrell, J. M. (1991). Effects of writing/speaking on comprehension of information for informed consent. *Western Journal of Nursing Research, 13,* 110-122.

Spiegelberg, H. (1984). *The phenomenological movement.* Boston: Martinus Nijhoff.

Staats, J. A. (1992). Chemical dependency. In J. H. Flaskerud & P. J. Ungvarski (Eds.), *HIV/AIDS: A guide to nursing care* (pp. 350-374). Philadelphia: W. B. Saunders.

Steel, E., & Haverkos, H. W. (1992). Epidemiologic studies of HIV/AIDS and drug abuse. *American Journal of Drug and Alcohol Abuse, 18,* 167-175.

Stein, E., Wade, K., & Smith, D. G. (1991). Clinical support groups that work. *Journal of Association of Nurses in AIDS Care, 2,* 29-36.

Stein, G. L. (1991). AIDS testing and the fault/no fault mentality. *Medical Humanities Review, 5,* 93-98.

Steinbock, B. (1992). The relevance of illegality. *Hastings Center Report, 22*(1), 19-22.

Stoddard, T. B., & Rieman, W. (1990). AIDS and the rights of the individual. *The Milbank Quarterly, 68,* 143-174.

Strauss, R. P., Corless, I. B., Luckey, J. W., van der Horst, C. M., & Dennis, B. H. (1992). Cognitive and attitudinal impacts of a university AIDS course: Interdisciplinary education as a public health intervention. *American Journal of Public Health, 82,* 569-572.

Stryker, J. (1989). IV drug use and AIDS: Public policy and dirty needles. *Journal of Health Politics, Policy and Law, 14,* 719-740.

Stuber, M. L. (Ed.). (1992). *Children and AIDS.* Washington, DC: American Psychiatric Press.

Swanson, J. M., Chenitz, C., Zalar, M., & Stoll, P. (1990). A critical review of human immunodeficiency virus infection—and acquired immunodeficiency syndrome-related research. *Journal of Professional Nursing, 6,* 341-355.

Tannebaum, J., & Butler, R. B. (1992). Reducing staff stress. *AIDS Patient Care, 6,* 21-24.

Tauer, C. A. (1989). The concept of discrimination and the treatment of people with AIDS. In E. T. Juengst & B. A. Koenig (Eds.), *The meaning of AIDS: Implications for medical science, clinical practice, and public health policy* (pp. 129-139). New York: Praeger.

Thiroux, J. P. (1986). *Ethics: Theory and practice* (3rd ed.). New York: Macmillan.

Torres, C. G., Turner, M. E., Harkness, J. R., & Istre, G. R. (1991). Security measures for AIDS and HIV. *American Journal of Public Health, 81,* 210-211.

Trenk, B. S. (1989). Hemophilia and AIDS. *AIDS Patient Care, 3,* 31-34.

Trianosky, G. (1990). What is virtue ethics all about? *American Philosophical Quarterly, 27,* 335-344.

Van den Boom, F. (1991). AIDS in the family. *AIDS Patient Care, 5,* 273-279.

Viney, L. L., & Bousfield, L. (1991). Narrative analysis: A method of psychosocial research for AIDS-affected people. *Social Science Medicine, 32,* 757-765.

Vladeck, B. C. (1989). The economics of a caring approach. In D. E. Rogers & E. Ginzberg (Eds.), *Public and professional attitudes toward AIDS patients* (pp. 85-95). San Francisco: Westview.

Wachter, R. M. (1992). AIDS, activism, and the politics of health. *The New England Journal of Medicine, 326,* 128-133.

Walters, L. (1991). Ethical issues in HIV testing during pregnancy. In R. R. Faden, G. Geller, & M. Powers (Eds.), *AIDS, women, and the next generation* (pp. 274-287). New York: Oxford University Press.

Watney, S. (1987). *Policing desire: Pornography, AIDS and the media.* Minneapolis: University of Minnesota Press.

Watson, J. (1990). Caring knowledge and informed moral passion. *Advances in Nursing Science, 13*(1), 15-24.

Webb, A. A., & Bunting, S. (1992). Ethical decision making by nurses in HIV/AIDS situations. *Journal of the Association of Nurses in AIDS Care, 3*(2), 15-18.

Wenger, N. S., Linn, L. S., Epstein, M., & Shapiro, M. F. (1991). Reduction of high-risk sexual behavior among heterosexuals undergoing HIV antibody testing: A randomized clinical trial. *American Journal of Public Health, 81,* 1580-1585.

Whitmore, G. (1988). *Someone was here.* New York: New American Library.

Wiggins, D. (1987). *Needs, values, truth.* Oxford: Basil Blackwell.

Wiley, K., Heath, L., Acklin, M., Earl, A., & Barnard, B. (1990). Care of HIV-infected patients: Nurses' concerns, opinions and precautions. *Applied Nursing Research, 3*(1), 27-33.

Williams, A. B. (1991). Women at risk: An AIDS educational needs assessment. *Image: Journal of Nursing Scholarship, 23,* 208-213.

Winick, C. (1991). Social behavior, public policy, and nonharmful drug use. *The Milbank Quarterly, 69,* 437-459.

Winslade, W. J. (1989). AIDS and the duty to inform others. In E. T. Juengst & B. A. Koenig (Eds.), *The meaning of AIDS: Implications for medical science, clinical practice, and public health policy* (pp. 108-116). New York: Praeger.

Wolf, S. M. (1992). Final exit: The end of argument. *Hastings Center Report, 22*(1), 30-33.

Wurzbach, M. E. (1990). The dilemma of withholding or withdrawing nutrition. *Image: Journal of Nursing Scholarship, 22,* 226-230.

Younger, J. B. (1990). Literary works as a mode of knowing. *Image: Journal of Nursing Scholarship, 22,* 39-43.

Zenilman, J. M., Erickson, B., Fox, R., Reichart, C. A., & Hook, E. W., III. (1992). Effect of HIV posttest counseling on STD incidence. *Journal of the American Medical Association, 267,* 843-845.

Zoloth-Dorfman, L., & Carney, B. (1991). The AIDS patient and the last ICU bed: Scarcity, medical futility, and ethics. *Quarterly Review Bulletin, 17,* 175-181.

Zuger, A. (1991). AIDS and the obligations of health care professionals. In F. G. Reamer (Ed.), *AIDS & ethics* (pp. 216-239). New York: Columbia University Press.

Index

About the Authors

Miriam E. Cameron, Ph.D., R.N., is a National Research Service Award Fellow in the School of Nursing, Center Associate for the Center for Biomedical Ethics, and Research Fellow for the Minnesota Area Geriatric Education Center at the University of Minnesota. She received her B.S.N., M.S. in nursing, and Ph.D. in nursing from the University of Minnesota. Focusing her doctoral study on bioethics, she conducted research and wrote a dissertation entitled *Ethical Problems Experienced by Persons With AIDS,* which is the basis of this book. This research was funded by a National Research Service Award from the National Center for Nursing Research at the National Institutes of Health (F31-NRO6327).

A former staff nurse, head nurse, nursing instructor, and nursing supervisor, she has been the recipient of numerous awards, scholarships, and fellowships. She has made presentations at local, regional, national, and international levels, and has published scholarly journal articles, a book chapter, and a book, *Hello, I'm God and I'm Here to Help You,* on topics about ethics and AIDS. Currently, she is conducting research, "Ethical Problems Experienced by Elders," funded by the National Center for Nursing Research at the National Institutes of Health (F32-NRO6808).

Edmund D. Pellegrino, M.D., is John Carroll Professor of Medicine and Medical Ethics, Director of the Center for the Advanced

Study of Ethics, and Director of the Center for Clinical Bioethics at Georgetown University. He received his B.S. from St. John's University and his M.D. from New York University. He served residencies in medicine at Bellevue, Goldwater Memorial, and Homer Folks Tuberculosis Hospitals, following which he was a research fellow in renal medicine and physiology at New York University. He has successively held the following positions: Founding Chairman and Director—Hunterdon Medical Center in Flemington, NJ; Professor and Founding Chairman—Department of Medicine, University of Kentucky; Founding Dean, Professor of Medicine and Vice-President of Health Sciences—State University of New York at Stony Brook; Chancellor and Professor of Medicine—University of Tennessee Center for the Health Sciences, Memphis; President—Yale-New Haven Medical Center and Professor of Medicine, Yale University; President, Professor of Philosophy and Biology—The Catholic University of America; and Professor of Medicine and Medical Ethics and Director—Kennedy Institute of Ethics, Georgetown University.

He is the author of more than 400 published items in medical science, philosophy, and ethics, and a member of many editorial boards. He is the author of *Humanism and the Physician* and coauthor with David C. Thomasma, Ph.D., of *The Philosophical Basis of Medical Practice* and *For the Patient's Good* and the founding editor of the *Journal of Medicine and Philosophy*. He is a Master of the American College of Physicians, Fellow of the American Association for the Advancement of Science, member of the Institute of Medicine of the National Academy of Sciences, and recipient of 38 honorary doctorates in addition to other honors and awards.